HeartBeats

By

Jef Huntsman

A Memoir

Heart Beats

This is a work of nonfiction, though most of the names and personal characteristics of the individuals involved have been changed to protect their privacy. Any resulting resemblance to persons living or dead is entirely coincidental and unintentional.

Jef R Huntsman

Copyright License Statement

Also, by the author
Jef Huntsman

Heart Attack, Yak, Yak

Tattered Portrait

Jamaica Rush
(A Carson thriller)

Bald Cats and Deaf Elephants
(A book of poetry)

Mosquito Sands
(A Carson thriller)

ACKNOWLEDGEMENTS

A hearty clap of the hands to my editor Kathy Jenkins and Diana Jensen who simplified things when my mind and typing fingers went astray as they do so often. A thunderous cheer goes to my wonderful writing friends, the scribes who poked and prodded me this way and that way. Their nagging was well heard, and I love how much better they made this book that is so dear to my heart. A special thanks to Harry Baldwin for his incredible cover work. Hugs and kisses to my wife, Diana, who stands by me when my incessant punch of the keyboard doesn't want to stop. And as always to my mom, Clara Wall Huntsman, whose full bookshelves always inspired me.

DEDICATION

This novel is dedicated to my son KYLE. He had more perseverance and happiness built into his young mind than I will ever have. He taught me compassion for others and how to gobble down a mountain of pills in one quick movement.

And to my father, James Keith Huntsman, an alignment and brake mechanic with a young, short-lived boxing career in prize fighting, who died on the operating table at the youthful age of 49 while undergoing one of the early versions of heart surgery. Thank you, Dad for all you taught me in my short fourteen years with you.

HeartBeats

By

Jef Huntsman

A Memoir

HEARTBEATS—PRELUDE THOUGHTS

This novel is about my cardiac arrest (at the relatively young age of forty-eight) and my son's brain tumor. But it's more than that. I'm sharing my story to help you find your own positive coping mechanisms during times of great tragedy. And holding on to the belief that things can get better.

We as humans seek ways to cope with disaster—the death of loved ones, loss of legs, debilitating diseases, or feelings of mortality. Some become depressed; others turn to alcohol, tobacco, drugs, food, or shopping—or a combination of these. Still others use work, books, television, hiking, or therapy, to name a few.

When disaster strikes, feeling bad about what life dealt you comes and goes but never truly leaves. Once my short-term depression eased, I used humor, laughter, smiles, and sarcasm to pull me from the reality that things in life are not always fair. Those gifts provided short, then eventually longer breaks from the thoughts of the tragedies that had struck me and Kyle. That alone gave me enough of a break to function and finally prevail over what had happened.

Think about this: one-third of my heart was nothing but dead, black muscle. I was given three to five years to live. Twenty years later, I'm still pounding in fence posts at my ranch and singing every morning.

Here's what that says to you: Never abandon hope. I yearn for you to come away from my story feeling better about yourself and your situation. Never forget that there is hope even in the most desperate of human trials.

Jef Huntsman

HeartBeats

1

The morning air thumped, and a fireball of Charmin tissue sailed across the sky. Our eyes followed the paper meteor as a black tail of smoke dropped ash like tiny parachutes feathering down from a burning plane. The flaming toilet paper finally dropped out of sight over the neighbor's cedar fence.

I glanced at my fourteen-year-old son. Kyle's eyes were as big as dinner plates.

He let out a long "Cooool!" as he held the black pipe above his shaved head. The stamped paw prints tattooed above his left ear glistened with a thin layer of sweat. The biggest smile I'd seen in some time spread across his cheeks, puffy from steroids.

"Grab the hose and follow me over there," I said.

Diana, my wife, shook her head as she stood watching, hands on hips and jaw muscles tight.

I picked up the bucket of water at my feet and ran around the snowball bush toward the neighbor's gate. Bursting through the gate, I saw a ball of flame in the middle of Mrs. Elan's rose bush. A patch of crusted snow in the shade of the fence reflected the flames. I doused the fireball with the water from the bucket just as Kyle came around the corner with a hose.

I tossed snow onto the remaining embers and carefully grabbed the wet, blackened mass of incinerated toilet tissue. Turning toward the gate, I noticed Mrs. Elan's glare above her crooked nose, pressed tight to the windowpane. Her skinny fingers gripped the window frame on the second story. I waved. She shook her head, scowled, and disappeared.

Kyle giggled as we headed back to our yard. "That was rad."

"Okay, time to run up and brush your teeth before we leave for school." I tossed the charred wad into the garbage can. "The glue on the barrel held this time, but we need to figure out why the roll catches on fire."

"The fire is cool." Kyle gripped the hose so tightly that his hands looked more like eagle talons. Water splashed across his Sketchers and darkened the rim of his denim pants. His muscles were having a hard time following orders from his tumor-infested brain.

"Only if were trying to burn Mrs. Elan's house down." I forced a smile.

"Yeah, she seemed ticked." He glanced up at the neighbor's window with a mischievous grin.

Most days started with the same old routine; *creatures of habit* was an apt description for us. But today was different. Both Kyle and I were jazzed by the early-morning cannon fire. As the euphoria wore off, I sat in the kitchen and realized I'd been woken up way too early. But the smile on Kyle's face was worth it.

As the sun tried to push through storm clouds, I began a slow stretch and twist of my shoulders, an outward push of my hands as I stretched my arm and hand muscles. *Wake up the body, and the mind will follow.* Of course, coffee would help. I poured 1 percent milk over some cereal and ate a slice of thinly buttered wheat toast while the wonderful aroma of percolating coffee filled the kitchen.

Kyle sat with me, downing his multi-colored cereal and orange juice. A stack of odd- shaped pills, some of them as big as grapes, were piled next to his plate. He talked about his "mean history teacher" and how the kids had played a joke on her. It seems she was furious after sitting down on a handful of tacks. Sputtered giggles turned into riotous laughter as the teacher used the words *sadistic* and *hell-bound delinquents* to describe the guffawing students. Kyle said that her red face looked like it was about to pop, and she furiously wagged her finger as she lectured for twenty minutes about "just punishment." Fortunately, said Kyle, the bell rang before her face exploded.

I looked over his math homework. It was fine except for a border of doodles on three sides. I advised him to doodle on a separate paper; Kyle acknowledged my advice but remained carefully evasive as he filled his backpack.

I finished breakfast, drank a second cup of my coffee, and headed for the shower.

I call it "my coffee" with great fondness of ownership, because I was the only one in the house who really enjoyed coffee. The others were amateurs; they drank things like milk and hot cocoa—drinks with no aroma, no flavor, and no personality. I had a long history with coffee; my mother had coffee every morning to perk her up and drank it again before going to bed to relax her. I smiled as I remembered the irony of those two opposite thoughts about what coffee did for her.

After my shower, I dressed and drove Kyle and a carpool of teens to school. They giggled and whispered and poked each other as I silently chaperoned. I returned home; I wasn't due at work for another ninety minutes.

I bounced up the entry stairs at my usual gait, arms extended like a long-distance runner. As I neared the top, agonizing pain shot through my back, radiating from my shoulders to my hips. The pain seared through my bones. I stopped mid-stride. *What the hell?* Not sure I could breathe at all, I managed to take in a shallow breath and hold it. Tears of agony filled my eyes. I carefully rounded the half wall of our split entry and eased over to the living room couch. My breath was distressed and purposeful. My eyes scrunched closed as a continuous shock of pain streamed through my entire body. I called out to my wife in a breathy moan that echoed in my head.

I couldn't find a comfortable position. Every robotic twist and turn brought on new agony. I bunched pillows at my side. I tried straightening my arms above my head in a stretch, my hands twisting, thinking my muscles were cramping. It didn't help. In fact, it made things worse. I stood up, extending my arms behind me and squeezing my shoulder blades together. I'm sure I appeared to be having some kind of bizarre seizure instead of struggling to relieve my pain. Regardless of what I tried, the constant torture kept spiraling up and down my back.

Diana came around the corner. "What's up?" Her carefree voice echoed happiness off the walls.

"I have . . . like . . . a . . . backache that's so painful." I paused between words as I tried to find them through the pain. "I don't know what I did." I moaned a little for emphasis, though I think my distress was obvious.

"You want an aspirin, or Tylenol, or something?"

"I don't . . . really know. Maybe . . . I'll just . . . lie down . . . on the couch here . . . see if it will go away. *Damn, shit, hell, every position hurts.*"

Diana looked at me with a sympathetic expression. I didn't swear often—only when I was too angry to form real words, or I was in great pain.

I hit the couch in a free fall, creasing the pillows. I tried to relax the pain away. I tried thinking of other things, pleasant things. I used contortion to work my back muscles. I took the aspirin Diana brought me with a cup of water and tried to relax. I tried to stay completely still and mentally coax my muscles into deep rest, a technique I had used in college to relax before a test. But the radiating pain I felt on the couch wasn't even close to what I had experienced before a college test. I couldn't seem to get rid of even the thought of the pain, let alone the reality. I needed a powerful sedative.

There I was—a hiker, a water-skier, a tennis player, a guy who was in great shape—immobilized by a backache. A silly backache.

I tried to figure out what I had done to mess up my back. I couldn't remember lifting anything heavy or turning wrong. But *they* say you can pull a back muscle simply picking up a piece of paper. *Hold on,* I thought. *I've picked up a lot of paper over the years and never hurt myself even a little.* I don't know who *they* are, but surely *they* are wrong on that one.

Diana called my work to let them know I would be late. I felt like a pitiful wimp, but the back spasm was so painful I couldn't even make that call myself.

Diana didn't want to go to work and leave me alone. I looked up at her. "Di, I pulled a muscle," I said through a contained grimace. "I'll be fine in an hour. Give the aspirin time to work." So, she left for work after asking if I needed anything else, leaving me to care for myself. It was Wednesday, November 16, 2000. That date would become permanently etched in my mind.

From my horizontal position on my soft pillows, I glanced through the window and watched her walk down the sidewalk to her car. It was a late fall morning. Five or ten leaves clung to each tree, holding on for a few more days until they drifted to the ground below, following the wind to the edges of the autumn bushes. Soon the snow would fall.

My forehead was covered with sweat. The deep, consuming pain in my back had drained gallons of energy. I took slow, deep breaths as I lay on one side, my back pressed into the semi-soft sofa pillows. Their sewn beaded edges cut into the nape of my neck.

The pain radiated in an ongoing cycle from my spine to my shoulders and down to the small of my back. It was relentless and seemed to have no point of origin. Every once in a great while, the pain receded for no more than a breath and then hit hard again.

I thought about that smiley face and its associated numbers displayed on charts in doctors' offices. The chart moved from a smiling face to one with a grimacing frown as the patient's self-described increments of pain increase. My pain on that sofa was *far* from the smiling face. In fact, I would have told a doctor my pain was at a twenty, even though the charts don't go that high. *Where is the chart for* this *kind of pain?*

I frantically grabbed the remote and clicked on the television. I needed sound. Something to drown out those stupid birds chirping outside the window. *General Hospital* came on. *Click.* Changed to *Family Feud. Click.* Switched to *Who Wants to Be a Millionaire. Click. Scooby Do. Click.* I decided to listen to the birds.

After going through various couch acrobatics, I found I felt better sitting up with a buttress of pillows bracing me. That seemed to work for a while. Later, I tried standing erect, in a C-shape like a geriatric, moving stoically around the room. I was a pathetic man in his forties who was imitating ninety—and doing it very well indeed. My back eventually felt better, but I became nauseous and unstable. I sat back down against the pillows.

I once read that if you have constant pain, you get used to it. It becomes the norm. I never wanted to reach that point.

After a couple of hours of pain interspersed with very brief episodes of relief and frequent torso twisting during which I unsuccessfully tried to find temporary comfort, I slowly moved the few steps from the couch to the kitchen cordless phone to call Diana. I had to collect myself, let a hard pain pass, and then push the buttons of hazily remembered numbers.

I told Diana I wanted to see a doctor—which for me was tantamount to admitting some sort of gross defect. She knew the pain must be bad for me to request a doctor. I hunched back onto the couch and put the cordless phone on the coffee table in front of the couch. Diana called back a few minutes later with an appointment three hours away. I wasn't sure I could endure that long, but I gave her a weak, panicked "Okay" over the phone. I mentioned she would have to drive me. It was the first time in my life I'd ever been so ill I couldn't drive myself.

The time dragged by. I listened to the ticking of the kitchen clock—and had I not been so sick, I would have torn its batteries out. Time seemed to pass even more slowly because of the excruciating pain. It's how I picture hell: suspended timeless years with unceasing physical misery. *Perhaps I should change my ways.*

I wasn't wearing a watch, and I was in too much pain to walk to the kitchen to check the clock. Pushing through my pain, I called Diana several times to find out how much longer before she was picking me up. I'm sure I sounded increasingly more pathetic with each call, and her voice appeared a little more on edge with each.

Diana's first answer was, "I'm picking you up in two hours, hon. Do you need to go to the ER instead?"

"Of course not." My pain was severe enough for the ER, but no internal organs or bones were protruding, and nothing green was spewing from my mouth. I figured a regular doctor visit would do.

After my many calls, Diana finally said, "I'm on my way; see you in ten minutes." I'm sure she thought I was being a crybaby over a pulled back muscle.

I am an on-time person. If I say I'll be somewhere at a certain time, I arrive with a few minutes to spare. Diana, on the other hand, runs on "Diana time." When she says, "I'm on my way," she normally means, "I'm finishing a few more phone calls, writing down a few notes, and then leaving the office." I was accustomed to that—and I knew her "ten minutes" could mean almost anything. That's usually no big deal, but my pain rendered me miserably distressed by the idea of Diana's "ten minutes." I simply hung on to the glimmer of hope that the pain would eventually end.

She arrived a few minutes later. Actually, I don't know how many minutes it took for her to get there. But at that point, it didn't matter.

2

The clinic was busy. Finding a parking stall even remotely close to the all-glass building was a feat. We traveled up and down rows of angled cars, searching with bobbing, quirky neck movements, like birds in a field searching for tidbits of food. We were always one aisle over when a stall opened, and each one closed quickly. I was too ill to be irritated. I was even patient, which was a big indicator that I didn't have a totally sound mind.

A parking spot finally opened relatively nearby; Diana hit the gas, swerving in front of and cutting off another vehicle. The driver waved at us vigorously with one finger, and I could read lips uttering colorful four-letter words. I smiled back. We had won. Our transmission was in park, and theirs wasn't.

When we got out of the car, it looked like we were about three blocks from the clinic doors. The distance faded in and out, as though it was on rails. But I knew my view was distorted by my pain, the same way some crazy people know they are crazy. Diana and I locked arms and moved toward the door; I let her direct me.

Once my insurance card was verified, designating me as worthy of health services, we sat down to wait. The selection of time-filling literature spread before us was limited to *Utah Health*, pamphlets about the colon, and a battered copy of an *US* magazine held tight ownership by a twenty-something girl. I did enjoy a few moments of peaceful time, staring at Nemo and friends in a large tank along the back wall. They seemed to just glide, in no hurry to end up anywhere. Their options were limited; they swam around the fake coral and past the bubbling treasure chest before doing it all over again. The fish seemed quite content, though, which was oddly calming for me.

The nurse called my name quickly enough that I hadn't even had time to play "What's Your Malady?" We had spent so many hours with Kyle in Utah and North Carolina hospitals that I can diagnose people in the waiting room with a fair amount of accuracy. The people with colds are easy: they clutch a tight wad of tissue, have a red nose, and have a wet hand. Every time they cough, they follow up by rubbing their hand on their pant leg. The flu is a little harder to detect; flu victims squirm in their chairs in an attempt to get comfortable. Sometimes they are stretched back, other times they resemble a curled-up snail.

People who are at the office for an annual checkup people seem calm, but there's often anxiety in their eyes. It's the *What If?* look. Kids who are there for immunizations are fine until Mom takes their hand and says, "Okay, the doctor is ready for us." Then all hell breaks loose. They likely imagine needles as long as corn stalks. Their tiny legs clamp to the chair legs unless they're making a panicked dash for the exit.

Sometimes I make up illnesses people might be afflicted with; one of my favorites is Hyperlabortosis, sick of too much work. The whole thing is quite a game, and it fills time in the waiting room with something other than reading those infected, used magazines.

But on this visit, there wasn't time. I didn't have the strength for the game, anyway. Every fiber seemed focused on my back pain.

Diana and I followed the nurse down one hall and up another. Except for short appendages and a small head, her dimensions matched those of a fifty-five-gallon drum. She walked with heavy, small steps. Her neck tilted slightly forward, like someone trudging up a hill with a backpack of rocks. She was winded by the time we stopped in front of a scale.

"Step up," she demanded, pointing at the scale. She had obviously worked at a U. S. Marine recruitment center before landing this gig.

"Should I smile?" I responded.

She gazed at me as though she was staring at a blank wall.

I tried again. "I hope you're not going to take my picture . . . I knew I would need a better shirt for this."

"Hardly," came her unamused, curt response. I decided she was basically a nonverbal type, but I felt a rapport growing, so I pasted a grand smile on my face. I was sure that would open her up.

But she was coy. She walked away without letting her smile show. Then she stopped and pointed through an open door. She followed me in with that same impassive bedside manner.

I couldn't wait for her to take my vital signs; from her pleasant manner, I knew she was going to try to distract me from my back pain. She pumped the blood pressure cuff until the pain relocated to my bicep. As she slowly released the pressure, I began breathing again. It worked. I forgot about my back pain. The barrel nurse asked why I was there, scribbling notes but acting like my answers were inconsequential to her.

The Barrel handed me a hospital gown and left the room without saying another word, shutting the door abruptly. She gave no instructions, though I'm not sure I needed any. Diana sat patiently clutching her purse.

"Personable!" I remarked to my wife.

"Yes, quite friendly." She agreed with a one-note laugh.

"I'm sure she's the employee of the month," I stated firmly with a nod of my head and a shrug of my shoulders.

"It must be hard for her to hold back like that," my wife quipped.

This banter went on for a while longer before the novelty wore off. We sat in silence. It felt good to be there, waiting for a cure. I was still in agonizing pain, but it took a back seat to the hope of being healed.

I began looking around the room. One wall boasted several paintings of clowns. One clown was juggling three poodles. Another was balanced on a beach ball. The final clown was posed upside down, his frizzy hair on the ground, tears on his cheeks, and his butt perched high in the air. All had various shades of sagebrush-colored hair. The opposing white wall featured medical illustrations of the eye and ear anatomy. A window gave a view of the traffic through bare winter branches. Medical instruments hung on the wall between the pictures.

With my ADHD personality, waiting has never been easy for me. I slid off the exam table in slow, tai chi movements. My breathing was raspy, and I felt like something discarded. I began checking out the magazines in the metal file holder on the counter. The selection was better in here than in the waiting room. However, after skimming anxiously through the magazines and watching traffic through slits in the blinds, I lost interest. Perhaps it was my head spinning; maybe it was my backache or my on-again, off-again fatigue. I needed stabilization. I sat down on the exam table. Then I lay down with my head on the sterile, covered pillow. Shooting pains circled my back, and I was dizzy. This exam room was no fun anymore.

Dr. Casper finally came into the room. His pale saurian face looked young and positive, not yet jaded by years of gazing at illness and disease every day. He had a long, slender nose; a thin, pointy chin; and receding, reddish-brown hair. His build was slightly slender and lean. He smiled at me and Diana with a mouth full of perfect teeth and eyes that radiated concern.

Dr. Casper read from my chart, looking up periodically to make sure we nodded in agreement as he read. Yes, I had back pain. Yes, it started this morning. No, I couldn't remember anything that had caused it. No, I had never before experienced back problems. No, I'm not on any medications. Saying that my vitals looked okay, he began examining me, asking me to tell him where I hurt. I was sore everywhere he pressed. I let out small gasps as he probed my back.

Finally, he stroked his chin and asked, "What were you doing when the pain started?"

"I was walking into the house after taking my son to school. This excruciating pain ripped across my back. I made it upstairs and sat down. That was it. I shoveled no walks, dug no holes—did nothing to yank my back out. I wasn't even in any hurry to get inside."

"Which muscles in your back started hurting first?"

"The left side mostly, but the pain seemed to take over my whole upper back, then move down to the lower. Then it radiated out so quickly that I couldn't tell a point of origin. Or maybe I was suffering too much to care. It has been excruciating."

"Is this sore here?" Dr. Casper asked, pressing his fingertips into my back again. "Or here?"

I winced. I even stopped breathing for a second. "Yes, but keep going, it's starting to feel good. Try a little to the left," I joked as a group of muscles tightened in a vise. I clamped my teeth and let out an unfamiliar noise.

"Are you okay?" the doctor asked.

I grimaced and nodded.

Dr. Casper gave a delayed chuckle as he added, "I am not a masseuse. You will have to refer to your wife for that treatment."

A doctor with a sense of humor. I like that, I thought.

"Oh, you're doing fine," I said. "We need this medical probing. Besides, she expects something in return. That washing hand thing."

Diana interrupted, "You mean, one hand washes the other?"

"Yeah, whatever," I said, changing to another painful position on the exam table.

I seemed to be conversing well, but on the inside, my teeth were ready to grind. My neck muscles were tight, and I was constantly searching for a position to lessen the pain in my back. I couldn't find one. I was stoic on the outside; on the inside, I wanted to scream or maybe just moan loudly for a bit. I'm sure my eyes looked like those of a discarded puppy look; we men try to be tough, but our eyes usually give us away.

Dr. Casper decided the pain must have been caused by influenza, bursitis, or some other similar thing. I was sent down the hall and given a blood test for influenza; after a short wait back in the exam room, we found out the test was negative. The doctor gave me muscle relaxants and painkillers to deal with the pain. With that, he sent on my way, expressing hope that the pain in my strained back would ease.

No one ever checked my heart. In fact, my heart was never even considered. Doctors are under pressure to make five-minute exams, coming up with a diagnosis and remedy within minutes. I take more time picking out fruit at the grocery store. Of course, I want cantaloupe that will last.

I slept in a drug-induced state that evening and throughout the next day. I may have read. I may have watched television. I may have danced in a skirt and heels on the backyard picnic table, but I don't remember. I cannot even recall arriving home.

Diana tells me I found refuge in the bed or on the couch, switching between them at four- to five-hour intervals while making eerie humming noises each time I changed. The pills did not seem to be doing anything more than giving me a headache.

Diana left for work late the next morning. She had one hearing regarding a restraining order and another in Farmington, an hour from her office in Holladay, Utah.

Nine months earlier, my son Kyle had been diagnosed with a brain tumor. The day after my backache, he was schedule for an MRI at 6 p.m., which he needed so he could start his new chemotherapy. Diana called me at 5:40, saying she was stuck downtown and needed me to drive Kyle to his hospital appointment. I felt like hardened crap. My back pains had worn me completely down; even my veins ached.

With little choice, I walked, hunched in agony, to the car and drove Kyle to the hospital. The drive took thirty minutes, and it took us five minutes to find the MRI room. Luckily, the doctor was waiting for us; they took Kyle right in, and the noisy machine started running.

I knew Diana was annoyed at me for complaining about having to drive Kyle to the hospital. I didn't blame her. Kyle's cancer was *much* more serious than my back problem.

Diana met me at the hospital shortly after I arrived. I was incredibly dizzy and lightheaded. My face white as copy paper. She told me later my speech was slurred. I told her I needed to go home. She tried to discourage me from driving, suggesting a cab or asking that I wait for her. She gave me numerous, unwanted options. I held my ground and said a weak, though stubborn, good-bye.

I drove home, able to pay only a minimal amount of attention to the road. My head floated in discomfort. I was on autopilot, fueled by pain pills and an obstinate male ego. In retrospect, I was incredibly lucky to pull into our driveway at the end of a safe trip. I inhaled deeply and exhaled with the same fervor. I stayed in the car for a few minutes, holding the steering wheel as pain shot through my back and waiting for my increasing dizziness to subside.

That second night, I recall eating bread and noodle soup. I was famished. I tried resting, but the back pain demanded constant attention. I took small bites, one after the other, as if on an assembly line. I recall struggling to breathe between bites and slurps. The food took my mind off the pain and I felt lethargic and hazy. My sitting would best be defined as slumped. I haven't owned pajamas since I was five, so my dress was a two-day-worn BOSE audio t-shirt, plaid boxers, and mismatched socks—one white, one blue. I followed myself to bed.

3

Rest and being zoned out on muscle relaxants eased my misery a notch. On a scale of one to ten, I was an eight instead of a twenty. I was just above roadkill on the feel-good meter. It was Friday, three days after I had seen the doctor.

Diana had to take Kyle to the hospital for blood tests and a lung function test at 1:00. She was amazing, trying to care for both of us. She was also lucky that only one of us complained, and it wasn't Kyle. I know the little trooper was also in torment, but he rarely showed it—always donning that funny sideways grin. I would like to be like Kyle, but I am such a great moaner that I truly hate to waste my talent.

Months later, Diana told me that she had complained to her secretary about me being such a pain in the ass over such a simple malady. She said they shared more than a few laughs about men being wimps, groaning over something as simple as a paper cut. She said she felt so bad when my flu/bursitis turned out to be a massive coronary.

Shortly after taking my morning pill, my back muscles responded ever so slightly. I didn't drink coffee. I couldn't remember ever before not drinking coffee. A shower seemed to help. Standing upright seemed to help. Bending over to put on my socks did not help. It made me slightly dizzy, feeling almost like a teenage hangover accompanied by acute distress. My eyes looked back at me from the mirror as if they were empty, lifeless sockets.

I had breakfast, more of a morning ritual than a need. I ate wheat toast, buttered lightly and spread with some strawberry jam someone had given us. I washed the toast down with a mini-can of V-8 and eight ounces of ice water.

I brushed my teeth with a light grip and a rubber arm. Gazing at my face in the mirror, saw a forty-eight-year-old man with ninety-three-year-old eyes. I washed my face again, rigorously massaging it with a rough hand towel to chase away the pallor and bring color back. After drying my face, I had a light-blue tint to my skin and a red, chapped nose. I was a horse of a different color. I looked again and told myself the mirror wasn't working.

Through my years, the worse I feel, the better I dress. I put on a light-blue shirt, never touched since coming back from the cleaner, who had pressed it into perfection with medium starch. I selected a tie with blue butterflies darting among brown water reeds. I felt queasy as I perused through my closet. The double-breasted, coal-black suit finished the look along with dress socks and polished black shoes. I didn't recheck the mirror. I wasn't sure the clothes could overpower the gray of my face, but I was hopeful.

My wife woke up. "Jef, what are you doing? You think you're getting ready for work?" She propped herself on one elbow. "You get back in bed!" She pointed directly at me.

"Really, it's been a long time since I was six years old. Are you my mother or my wife?"

"If you're childish enough to think you can go to work, then I must be old enough to be your mother."

My chin tilted up in defiance. "Really!"

"The suit looks great, but YOU look like shit. You're hunched over, your eyes are swimming in prescription pills, and your face is gray."

"Really!"

"And you seem to have lost your vocabulary. Go take off the suit and get some rest."

"Really! . . . Besides, I feel fine. I rested last night. It didn't work. By the way, what I need is called *sleep,* not *rest*; maybe you've heard of it." I pointed two fingers back at her.

"You feel fine because those pills have relaxed every muscle in your body. Unfortunately, they've apparently done double duty on your brain."

"Really!"

"There's that word again!"

"I need to go to work. I feel much better. I think work would be better than watching the bedroom blinds not move for another thrilling day."

"You feel better?" she said sarcastically, her head bobbing. She sat up and pointed her long finger again. "Okay! Bend over and pick up that small stool and put it on the other side of the room as quickly as you can."

"Uhhh, what? Am I your cabana boy?" My head swam across another wave of nausea.

"You are if you want to go to work today." She rubbed her chin, smiled, and kept pointing from the stool to the other side of the room like a damn windshield wiper. She has always been beyond persistent—a Type A personality trying to boss another Type A. What a combination.

"Well, not that you can stop me from going to work; but all right." With elbows stretched out and hands on hips in defiance a powerful spasm surged through my back. I turned my head away from Diana's sight to wince.

I bent over, using my knees as much as possible, picked up the stool, and moved it to where she kept pointing with her finger. Pain shot through my entire body. Bile almost erupted from my stomach. It was even harder putting the stool down than it had been picking it up. On the outside, my face, sallow as it was, tried to show the whole endeavor as a simple act. On the inside, my teeth were clenched like a vise about to break. I was sure I would need dental work after my show of willpower.

After catching my breath, I slowly forced out the words, "See, I'm fine."

"Did you fool yourself?" Her mouth briefly tightened in a line. "Even though that was quite a performance, you didn't fool me. And the Oscar goes to . . ." She held her palm out toward me, "the cabana boy."

She snickered, then a serious expression crossed her face as she watched me where I stood defiantly. "Let's see if you can move it back."

"I don't need these games. I admit I will have to take it a bit easy, but I'll be just fine."

"You are stubborn."

"And healthy!"

"You're going to scare the employees."

"Yeah, they won't dare call in sick, after they see me rise from the grave." I laughed weakly.

Diana did not see the humor. Her eyes rolled, she dropped to her pillow, and pulled the covers over her head.

Stupidity is a male art form.

Driving to work—medicated, with sensitive eyes and back pain—was a challenge. I should have thought of those warnings on the pill bottle: *Do not drive or operate heavy machinery after taking this prescription.* That sounds great when you're sober or nonmedicated. Under the influence, though, that statement doesn't even come to mind. At least I wasn't going to operate heavy machinery. I believed at the time that my jeep Cherokee would be listed under light duty. It was definitely smaller than a road grader.

I made it to work and got out of the car all right. I amazed myself by making it to the front door and then to my desk. However, I felt as though I was breathing sand and trudging through mud.

The desk was moving. The room was tilting on an axis. Everywhere I looked I saw blurriness and chaos. Most things I tried to focus on were pulsing. The whole environment felt wrong. I clung to my chair for support and safety. My hands moved slowly and carefully from the chair to a firm hold on the desktop. The sensation reminded me of the time I got off an amusement ride and held on to a stranger's shoulder and a park bench before erupting stomach acid and chewed popcorn into a well-tended flower bed.

This time my stomach was hanging in there, but my head was having those same flushing waves of nausea. In time, I started to feel better. I took deep, full breaths of stale indoor air. It was uplifting, in a dusty, coffin-like way.

I had arrived at the office early. The sales crew began to arrive. Everyone was asking if I was okay or commenting about my pallor. Any person with a lesser ego would have been crushed. I figured they were just being concerned. I also didn't feel well enough to care about the pitying looks that passed in reverence as if I was displayed in a box and surrounded by flower arrangements in the front of a room lined with pews.

I spent the next three hours doing absolutely nothing. The clock was the only thing in my office with any movement. Well, to be accurate, I did alternate between holding on to my desk, gripping the arms of my chair, and rolling a pen in my fingers with enough force to squeeze out ink. Finally, I tried standing. I got up an inch at a time while grasping the edge of the desk and cautiously adjusting to the change in altitude.

As I stood, I realized at once I needed a bathroom break. My bladder was extremely full, and the sensation came on me without warning. My legs instinctively took on the movement of closed scissors, a stop-the-flow maneuver. I held that ludicrous position for a few moments. Dizziness hit from the quick motion.

The nausea eventually subsided. I moved as quickly as I could to the nearest men's room and stood with adolescent glee in front of the porcelain goddess. A deep breath of finished satisfaction and the goodness of everyday events pumped my spirits as I washed my hands. It had been a brief period of normalcy. It felt good.

That illusion evaporated when I caught a glimpse of my new look in the splattered bathroom mirror. I was blue—no, I was more blue-green. I looked a little like a turtle in a fancy shell. I was dressed for *Gentleman's Quarterly* but had an off-color head that resembled a plucked, blue-green chicken. I looked worse than when I left the house—an unbelievable feat. I had to hold my breath as my back pain increased. My brow dropped hard on frightened eyes.

"Woooaaaa!" I bellowed.

I turned and stumbled toward my office. As I moved along the carpeted path, two people commented, "You don't look so good," and one asked, "Jef, are you all right?" If they were trying to build up my self-esteem, they were a tad off. I was feeling disillusioned enough without their comments.

It took a stretch of nonexistent power to walk to my windowed office. It was as though I was watching myself move instead of actually moving. I finally made it and collapsed in the swivel chair. The seat gave softly against my weight. The chair gave little comfort to my state of being, but it was an accomplishment to arrive.

The secretary stared at me from five feet away. Her sparsely tinted lips moved as the sound of her voice traveled slowly in my direction. "Jef, you need to go home, or maybe to a hospital. You don't look so good."

I felt terrible. I couldn't even look up without getting shaky. Stupid mirror.

When I didn't respond, she asked, "Do you want me to give you a ride?"

I was consumed by my body's adjustment to feeling completely exhausted and loose while being enveloped with pain. In retrospect, I'm pretty sure I was in and out of consciousness.

I was later told that I sat staring at my desk, my hands flat on it. I was also told that I didn't respond for several minutes, my face turned blue, and that I had a lost, vacant look in my eyes.

After what seemed like an eternity, I came out of it. I blinked hard several times and scrunched up my face in response to my secretary shaking my shoulder. I looked at her face, and in a moment of clarity, I knew I shouldn't be there. I realized I should have stayed home. My wife was right! Damn!

In slow motion, I punched the number one on my cell phone—the number that connects me to my wife. She is usually on her phone at work, and I usually have to talk have to her secretary or leave a message. That day the stars were aligned: she answered her own phone before I had to leave a message.

In a tone not much louder than a whisper, I told Diana to pick me up and take me to the doctor. Any doctor. *Now!*

A few minutes later, she called back after checking with the doctor's office. I was still slightly mesmerized, staring at the surface of my desk. The phone jarred me back to reality.

Though I could detect some worry, her voice sounded business-like. "We have an appointment in a half hour with a Dr. Martini. I'll be there in ten. Wait by the front door."

She waited for me to respond, and finally asked, "Are you there?"

"Yeah, I'll meet you out front. Sorry . . . I'm a little slow today."

"I'll hurry!"

I was surprised when she hung up. I expected her to say something like, *I told you it wasn't a good idea for you to go to work.* But she didn't. There was no gloating at all. I knew then that I was quite ill.

I looked up at Janelle, my secretary, as if I wanted to say something, but my thoughts were too slow to organize. It was as though time was drifting by languidly, but only about ten minutes had passed.

Janelle interrupted my floating thoughts. "Get your coat on and go! I'll take care of things here." As always, she was being helpful and kind, and I was unable to even express my gratitude. A thank-you smile lingered just behind my lips. It wouldn't form, but I knew she understood.

4

Diana dropped me off at the front door of the clinic with instructions fit for a five-year-old. I thanked her. I had nothing in me, no smart-ass comeback. *I truly must be sick.*

The door was weighted, and I was scarcely able to open it. Right behind me was a pretty, bulky woman with a tribe of elementary-aged children; I held the door open as they each entered. They scurried by, looking scared, glancing furtively with wide eyes at the man with the greenish-blue face. Bringing up the rear, the woman nodded at me, flashed an infectious smile, and thanked me for my help. I felt a responsive grin on my face, the first of the day. As I watched her and her ducklings stroll away, I decided she was either a schoolteacher on a field day or the original octo-mom.

The clinic personnel had approved my last-minute appointment was because I was out of pain pills and was suffering intensely from what I thought was influenza or possibly bursitis. The nurse explained that the doctors there could not rewrite another physician's prescription without personally seeing the patient. My physician, Dr. Casper, was off for the day. When Diana explained that I couldn't make it through the weekend in this much pain, the clinic nurse adjusted the schedule to fit us in before the weekend. While the pain pills took only a slight edge off, I was thankful for even that sliver of help. I couldn't imagine enduring the weekend without them.

Diana had caught up with me. The waiting room was sparsely filled; we must have arrived during a lull in the sickness parade. Entering the exam waiting room with the speed of a slug, I realized there was a vast void in my mind. Mama duck was filling out paperwork while her little ducklings stared at the fish tank. We hardly creased the cushions on the chairs before the nurse called my name.

As Dr. Martini checked this and that, my wife told him about my last few days. I was mostly a bystander at this point. I don't normally like being talked about, as though I am not there, but I was passive for once.

The doctor checked my heart. Had me take deep breaths and exhale. He lifted my eyelids and peered at them. He checked my reflexes and lymph nodes. I stayed quiet and hoped he could fix whatever was wrong with me.

After ten minutes of robotic probing and conversation about me, the doctor sent me to have blood drawn and to have some chest x-rays. I held Diana's hand, staggering in an incoherent stride as she led me to the right area. I faded in and out of consciousness as pain hit in waves.

The phlebotomist in the lab had the mannerisms and wide-open eyes of too much coffee following an all-night cramming session. She eyed my arms with the pleasure of a vampire. I am one of those people whose arms display a road map of translucent blue veins barely below the surface my skin. She had no trouble poking a vein; with relaxed effort and quick agility, she filled two tubes of blood, pressed a cotton ball firmly against the puncture wound, and taped it down.

She pointed across the hall to the x-ray sign, saying, "Your next stop."

My lips parted for the automatic thank-you but thought better of it, sucking my lips tightly against my teeth. *Thank you for sticking a needle in me and taking out my life-giving blood.* What was I thinking? I blankly looked across the hall.

The eight-by-five x-ray waiting area held two light-colored, oak chairs; an empty table resembling a heavy, painted, upside-down crate, and bare walls. The chairs were rigid and uncomfortable, but I was so exhausted I didn't care. To me they seemed soft and comfortable. I slumped down, trying to relax, my feet stretching almost to the other side of the room.

A gourd-shaped tech ventured out of a cylindrical, black door, holding what appeared to be large, plastic sheets. I hadn't even noticed the door. He promptly attached the sheets to a white screen. Flipping a switch on the side of the screen, he stood attentively. His head shook up and down in an affirmative manner as if he had a tremor. It was the oddest nod I had ever seen.

The Gourd pointed at a door marked *X-Ray Room* and said, smiling, "You're next."

I looked around the small, empty room with a questioning look on my face. I gestured with my hands, as though others were in the room. He ignored me. My wife smacked my arm.

Rubbing my arm as though it was in terrible pain, I whispered, "I may be sick, but I still like to have fun."

Diana tilted her head, giving me a threatening, negative scowl. But I couldn't help noticing her irrepressible half-smile.

I whispered again. "Remember, I'm the patient; careful with the arm, Mohamed Ali." When she didn't respond, I waited a few beats then said, "Seriously, I really do feel like crap."

I stood with my shirt off and my hands in the air while the Gourd maneuvered the x-ray cartridge. He grabbed me by my shoulders and adjusted my position slightly. A big machine pointed directly at me. He went behind a wall with windows and told me to hold my breath. There was a noise, and we were done with that view.

I was rearranged for a side view, held my breath, and another noise ground out from the machine.

After looking at my x-rays, he said there was a problem with one. The Gourd had me repeat the side view. After looking at the picture on the screen for a few minutes, he nodded; it may as well have been a masterpiece to him. I saw no difference in the two films. Diana thought she did. I thought she was flirting with the Gourd—if she was, I was too sick to care.

On the way back to the exam room, I kept wondering why I had thanked the Gourd for taking the x-rays. It was nothing more than polite gibberish, which I typically avoid. I felt so congenial. I really was ill, and it was something to which I was unaccustomed.

We impatiently waited a short time for Dr. Martini to return; Diana and I stared at the walls, the sink, each other. We said nothing. Our faces were blank except for a rising of the eyes signaling, *What now?* As we both blew out sighs of exasperation, there was a knock on the door.

Dr. Martini came in with my x-rays, my patient file, and numerous papers under his arm. He threw them on the counter by the sink.

"Jef, we've checked your blood and x-rays." There was a brief pause. "You have had a heart attack. I've verified this with another physician. It also appears you may have pericarditis."

Diana and I both nodded our heads robotically in agreement, as though we had been told by a maître de that our table would be ready in a moment. The nodding seemed to go on for minutes. I had no sarcastic come-back. The doctor continued talking, but we were both stuck on two words he had said.

Suddenly reality hit. Diana and I became immobile. The doctor stopped talking. I fastened my eyes onto hers for what seemed like centuries. I stopped breathing. My body was rigid. The loudest noises in the room were the whooshing of air through the vents and people whispering behind the door.

I finally took a breath and shifted my weight on the chair. Diana and Dr. Martini turned to me, as though I had said something. I shifted my weight to the other leg. The silence seemed to last forever.

After a guttural noise that bounced off the walls, Dr. Martini cleared his throat and said, "You need to go to an emergency room, *now*."

I looked at Diana. She looked stunned, and that was a new expression for her. She always had an opinion, something to say. At the moment, she had nothing.

I gazed back at Dr. Martini without much acknowledgment.

"Is there a hospital you would prefer?" he asked. "Saint Mark's is probably the closest, and they have excellent cardiac care."

Diana started to say something, but my lips finally parted, interrupting. "Heart attack, like a . . . real . . . heart . . . attack?"

"Yes," Dr. Martini said, "It obviously happened a few days ago, but you need to get to an emergency room!"

I stretched my neck, as though waking up. "Wow!" was all I could think to say.

"What should we do?" Diana asked.

"I could call an ambulance, or you could drive there yourself; whichever you choose, it needs to be now," Dr. Martini said.

"So," I hesitated, "it never was a backache or flu?"

He said nothing but looked at me with sadness. I understood.

With a distraught look on her face and force in her voice, Diana interjected, "Let's go. I'll drive. Or would you rather have an ambulance ride?"

I turned toward the doctor. I had gained a little of myself back. "The way she drives, we'll be there before you can dial up the ambulance." I held my chest firmly with my right hand. The reality was settling in. I began to understand things I did not want to know. Fear struck, and I gave a humorless laugh.

Diana grabbed my arm with urgency.

I wasn't finished. Turning back to the doctor, I said, "You should ask our kids what cows and telephone poles look like at a hundred miles per hour."

I didn't even mind being led away as I was pulled and forced down the hall. Dr. Martini followed, handing Diana the x-rays. She grabbed them in her free hand.

Before turning the corner, we both sang, "Thanks" over our shoulders.

"I'll call, so they'll expect you and will take you right in," Dr. Martini said.

We hurried down the last corridor and didn't look back.

We strapped in and were off. I murmured, "Heart attack." I thought it was only in my mind, but a repeated whisper escaped unthinkingly.

As the car jolted, I immediately became best friends with the arm rest. Holding on tightly to something soft and inanimate gave me comfort. My triceps contracted as my fingers grasped the door handle and seat cushion. I focused on both hands as we maneuvered the streets at double the posted limit. Oddly, I was totally relaxed. Except for normal autonomic functions, like breathing, few neurons were firing.

The doors of the emergency entrance whooshed open at our arrival. I was being pampered by my love, Diana. That was nice. It was caring. Though still stunned by my diagnosis and locked in deep thought about my own prognosis, I enjoyed the attention but knew that it would get old fast.

5

I urinated orange into the institutional, stainless-steel bowl. Heart disease had rendered me incapable of much more than automatic functions. A face of greenish-gray rubber attached precariously to my skull stared back at me from the wall. I was bewildered, my mind fading in and out on rusty hinges.

I began coming out of the low-blood-pressure haze. I startled as I stared at the surprising color flowing forcefully into the toilet bowl. I was fascinated and confused at the deep, dark orange. I tried to blink it away. Nope, still there. It was as if I had drunk an Apollo amount of Tang—it was a weird color, orange with a hint of red. I watched intently for the color to change back to a weak-tea amber. Any similar shade would do. Standing immobile, I dripped the last couple of orange drops and zipped up. I didn't notice if the lid was up or down. Did I bull's-eye it, or had my aim returned to childhood meandering? I had little clue. My mind stayed focused on the orange liquid in the bowl. As I reached for the flush handle, I retreated. I needed evidence.

Exhausted and dull, I robotically did an about-face, washed my hands, and turned the faucet off. I had just enough cognition to know I needed to share this orange problem. The pee was disconcerting. My mind wavered between knowing and not quite sure. *Hallucinations?* I took a minute to figure out where I was and why I was there. I never completely resolved the dilemma. The tile stared with square white eyes back at me. I headed to the door like a lost drunk, inebriated from a faulty heart, orange urine, and fear.

The wooden door was heavy. Pushing with strength I barely had, I entered the noise and smells and glare of the ER. As I took a step forward, Diana appeared at my side. Like warm vapor, I felt her presence before she grabbed my elbow and guided me toward my curtain. I don't know if I needed her help, but it felt good and right.

I licked my lips to speak. "It's all orange—dark orange."

She had a bewildered look; her brow scrunched and then relaxed. "Your face? No, your face is gray. You look . . ." She paused. Her hands rubbed my shoulder. "What's wrong?"

"No, my urine, it made the toilet orange."

"Orange?" It was a question, pronounced slowly with each letter emphasized the way one talks to someone who can't speak your language. And louder, because obviously, if it's louder, I would understand it better. She tilted her head, looking puzzled. "An orange toilet? You're seeing things." She dipped her head and scrunched the skin between her eyes with the last two words of her question.

"Please go look," I said. "I didn't flush, because I wanted someone to see. It's like the fruit, only darker. I had a heart attack. I'm dizzy, disoriented, and I walk slowly. But my mind is fine. I peed orange. It doesn't seem—right." I knew things were hazy, but I'd seen exactly what I said I'd seen. I wasn't sure if the hospital gown was open in the back, though I held on to enough reality to understand that I wasn't sure. At least, I was 75 percent sure.

"Okay . . . okay. Let's get back to the bed," she whispered, trying to soothe me and guiding me back to my gurney by the elbow, like one guides children back to their beds.

An ER nurse waited with other-things-to-do tolerance, hands on hips. A comfortable posture for her. A tech waited to her right, at attention, appearing to count ceiling tiles.

"That is not a bed," I protested weakly, pointing to the narrow mattress. There were rails and electronic buttons and wheels the size of a Frisbee.

Halfway there, I stopped, trying to recall if I had washed my hands, running through faucet sounds and towel movement in my mind. I turned to Diana saying, "I can't remember if I washed my hands. Stop for a minute. I need to catch my breath. my head's spinning."

Diana recognized my dilemma, "Your hands are still holding the paper towel." We stopped while I caught my breath my heart rate lowered. It didn't take long.

"Oh, yeah. Here." I handed her the wadded paper. This heart problem was incredibly frustrating. I wanted my old heart back—the good one. I needed the one from my college years that celebrated in happy tempo when I aced a test.

I tried to exert a fleeting amount of personality, smiling at the nurse waiting in my curtained ER space. The machines beeping, the rigid gurney, and the nose-biting smells all seemed inviting in an absurd, sanitary way. I held my breath as a sharp pain burst down my spine hard enough to shatter it into pieces.

The agony subsided.

"They're here to take some blood or something." Diana glanced over for confirmation from a thin nurse. "Can we help you up on the gurney?"

"Just take your time," said a lean lady with a stethoscope hanging like a broken necklace around her slight neck. The nurse was young with such a deep tan that she looked like an overcooked, bronze string bean. Her arms and neck were all gristle and cords. The neck cords branched out to bony shoulders that poked through her flowered scrubs. Her face was kind and wind-worn, reminding me of a picture of a hundred-year-old Navajo I had once seen. Pale red lipstick curved in a smile that was surprisingly comforting.

I eased over toward the edge of the bed.

"This is me walking fast. You don't have to wait up." I was surprised I could still crack jokes.

"You're doing fine," Pale Red Lipstick encouraged.

I looked at my feet, sliding and pausing, sliding and pausing. "So, this is fine?"

"After the trauma your heart went through, yes."

Lethargically crawling onto the ER bed, I reclined and let my body relax. The nurse hooked me back up to all the necessary beeping, buzzing, and inflatable cuff machines. The doctor arrived.

My new, and only, cardiologist appeared to be in his early forties, with happy yet concerned eyes and a learned brow.

Thick, brown, curly hair covered the top of his ears. His hair was neither combed nor out of place, but plainly natural and flowing, like a well-watered thick shrub. Stubby fingers connected to athletic arms and a slightly softened torso. He had no Band-Aids or scars on his fingers—no tattoos of sinking ships on his arms. I took that as a positive sign. The things that distinguished him as a doctor were a name tag, a take-charge manner, and the stethoscope draped around his neck. Oh, and that noble, caretaking stance.

Lying in my curtained bedroom, I explained to both him and the nurse my concern and amazement over my new pee color. I told them I hadn't flushed. I assured them I did wash my hands (I assumed they were as concerned as I had been about that). I told them that orange pee had never come out of me before, and it didn't seem right. I didn't want to pee again until it was fixed.

But the doctor only wanted to check my heart. I kept pushing the orange urine issue until they seemed to almost wonder if it were true. But they were skeptics.

"You can't touch me until you check the toilet," I said, recoiling from their touch as much as I could.

"Please. He won't stop about this," Diana pleaded.

The nurse and the doctor exchanged glances.

The cardiologist and the nurse went with Diana to check out the offending color. They all agreed it was deep orange. The doctor decided the color had nothing to do with my heart. In his opinion, it was "not a problem," but he promised to have someone from the urology clinic visit me.

My fear swelled like an ocean wave. Not only did I now have a cardiologist, but I also needed a urology specialist. My body was like a puzzle with pieces scattering at the slightest nudge.

"Your heart is our main concern at this point," said the cardiologist.

The cardiologist, Dr. Vandoven, asked me to put nitroglycerine tablets under my tongue. They were supposed to help ease the pain. They did not. They only made me lightheaded.

Later, after realizing my teeth were clasped in a grinding lock of misery, they gave me morphine for the pain. The morphine nauseated me while my pain level still hovered above ten on the smiley-face chart. I preferred the pain.

I was exhausted. The thought of the orange situation had brought me out of my cardiac stupor. I looked at Dr. Vandoven. "So orange is not a problem—but it *is* abnormal, right?" I truly needed some type of confirmation on that. For me, the heart thing wasn't as blatant as my personal dye job in the toilet.

"Your heart condition is the immediate difficulty," said Dr. Vandoven. "But yes, your urine does have an odd color. Just relax and rest. Let us work on the major problem—your heart."

I had a heart attack at forty-eight years of age, my urine is orange, I'm exhausted from pain and sleepless nights, my breathing is shallow and hurts, this is the first time I have ever been a patient in a hospital, and I'm somehow supposed to rest? Oh, yeah, and now I'm a person with a cardiologist. A chill screamed through my muscles.

My doctor could tell what I was thinking. He patted my forearm. "I know this is a lot to take in, but your heart needs you to relax for it to recover," he said sternly, in that no-nonsense tone doctors use.

"I'm not going home tonight, am I?" I questioned foolishly, knowing I what the answer would be while hoping they had simply misdiagnosed me, and I really had something simple like a toothache or a pulled tendon.

"Not likely." His firm voice was tinged with a touch of humor, as if I'd made a joke. "They're going to run some tests, and I will check back periodically. Quit worrying about the urine. Your heart is the primary concern. We'll look at anything else after we have more information on your heart. Does that sound okay?"

"Fine, but if my pee is orange, what color is my blood?" I said, nodding my head, which only made me lightheaded and sick to my stomach. *It's hard to be a smart-ass and so damn sick at the same time.*

"Jef, just relax and keep your head down on the pillow," Diana said, in an attempt to shut me up.

"That's another thing. This isn't a pillow. It deflates where I my head is and billows where it isn't."

Diana looked at me, took in a soft breath, and said, "Do you want me to get another pillow?"

"No. I'm just not very good at being sick. I haven't had a lot of practice. Give me some time and more meds. I'll mellow out."

The entire time Dr. Vandoven talked to me, he held my shoulder and looked directly at me. I had just met him, but I trusted him. He didn't give me false promises. He described facts as he knew them. He took time to answer my questions. He laughed at my sarcasm. Dr. Vandoven had the ability to convey genuine concern, even after years of seeing patients. I had only seen that in a few of the physicians I had worked with during my college years as a scrub tech at the University Medical Center. Most of the interns had that deep concern for the human condition, but most of them lost it after a few years of handling the sick and afflicted. Dr. Vandoven was one of those rare, immediate friends with whom you have rapport after a just brief conversation. Yes, I trusted my new doctor very much.

Dr. Vandoven walked away without answering my question about the color of my blood. I guess it could have been taken as rhetorical, though deep in my mind I didn't think it was. He looked a bit amused as he glanced back at me before rounding the corner.

I lay back on the ER gurney. I was suddenly satiated with tiredness and anxiety, falling in and out of sleep. A parade of insertions, proddings, and x-rays began that would continue for hours.

* * *

I blinked a few times. I was still in the ER suffering from unacceptable orange pee, and a heart thrown out of whack.

Here I was in a big room with all the other off-the-street cases. I hadn't been evaluated thoroughly enough to be admitted to my own room yet. My hospital stay was still in the beginning stage. I hardly even felt mistreated yet—but there was still a lot to unfold, a lot of skin to be poked, a lot of chest hair to be ripped off with EKG adhesive pads, an abundance of pharmaceuticals to ingest.

I tried to relax. I was perched on a three-inch-thick slab of foam encased with black, washable vinyl. Covering the black vinyl was a hospital-white sheet fitted at the corners. As I started to relax, my mind wandered and considered absurdities and inconveniences. My heart attack was the biggest inconvenience. It was something hard to hold, inspect, and understand. The heart attack gave birth to other inconveniences—IV hookups, my body being inspected and poked, dizziness, being cared for like an helpless infant, and gurgling of my injured heart that I could feel in my chest. Being immobile was one of the hardest inconveniences of all.

Everyone pushed me to *take it easy,* as if I was home relaxing with a good book and a glass of red wine. No way. I couldn't sleep on this antiseptic-smelling sheet. I kept envision it being washed hundreds of times in caustic chemicals that stripped away the blood and urine, sweat and skin cells, Betadine and drool, and other pieces of human suffering and illness. This one sheet had probably been under burn patients, cancer patients, motorcycle trauma patients, fungus-infested patients, broken arm patients, children with head lice and runny noses, patients with bladder retention problems, elderly patients sucking in their last breaths, and birthing mothers. All forms of human frailty and economic status had laid their sweaty backs on those rewashed sheets. Groans of pain had been imbedded in the weave of the fabric. My logical mind wanted to believe my brighter-than-white, clean sheet was sterile, but reality made me want to levitate just above the mattress. It was one more thing to keep me awkwardly stirred up, far from relaxed.

Hopefully, fatigue would win over, and my eyes could close without being haunted by years of imagined sheet stains. As I looked a little closer mat the sheet, I noticed a couple of faded, gray spots that I wasn't too sure about. I slid a few inches away from them and tried to look at something else.

I closed my eyes and tried to relax. I listened to my breathing. Relaxation happened in spurts and sputters. The reality of the recent heart attack kept my senses on slight edge. Each inconsequential noise pulled me toward it.

As most patients know, hospitals have little to do with rest. It seems there is a conveyer belt of staff and machines circling like buzzards, pecking at your bones. They sit you up, turn you, examine you, and prod you. Wheelchairs run you here and there, taking you to room-sized machines that beep and squeal while everyone else stands behind a safety barrier. Your vanity swirls away like waste being flushed down the toilet. Self-respect vanishes as you are surveyed in places and ways only a degenerate would consider. Rest comes only from prescriptions that you find yourself praying for.

In the next few days I would learn more about hospitals and patient care than I ever wanted to know.

Hospitals specialize in forced recuperation. There are pills to take and interns to enlighten. Nurses wake you up to make sure you are sleeping. Machines continuously beep and hum; some spit out paper like crickets chirping. Floor polishers spin on a hard surface; there is laughter and crying in the distance. Mops whish and metal pans fill up with all sorts of vile liquids ejected from the human body. Ladies in heels sound like Clydesdales on a corrugated tin roof. Visitors with obnoxious, loud voices tell hospital stories that would scare even a healthy person.

Then there are the interrogation lights that are flipped on and off, and on and off again, while hospital personnel check this, that, and the other. But don't forget, there's always that one light with the hidden switch that's on twenty-four/seven, making complete darkness impossible. I have wondered if all those distractions are the reason patients need sleeping pills and pain medication in the hospital.

And what about the people you call friends and family? Just when your eyelids start to droop and your body has arrived at the edge of rest, visitors show up with balloons and carnival acts. They say things like, "You look terrible," and, "How do you feel?" They turn on the television because they're bored, and they sit on the edge of your bed to comfort you. Visitors accidently pull tubes that are adhesively attached to red skin and short hairs. Visitors stay too long and bring in food you can't eat. *I have coronary artery disease; could you please bring me a super-size order of fries, dripping with foul, perfidious fat?* They put pollinating plants all around the bed that provoke your allergies, and the smell makes you wonder if you're already at your funeral. If you are lucky enough to finally fall asleep, you'll invariably wake up with everyone whispering in a soft roar. They impose their thoughts about related and irrelevant illnesses and medical care until you wish you had the strength to put a closed fist to their jabbering jaws.

Time out: I should be fair here. I have a split personality about guests. When I wasn't feeling well, visitors were annoying. But when most of the pain subsided, I enjoyed their visits. They were heartwarming and encouraging. I enjoyed them most after I left the hospital. During my hospital incarceration, I was medicated enough and anxious enough that I just wanted to be left alone. Once I was in better health, my visitors were anointed saints.

Back to our regularly scheduled programming: this was the first time I'd been hospitalized, but I was learning quickly. As I tried following my doctor's advice, I couldn't help thinking, *I need to get out of here, go home, and close the bedroom door.* It is no mystery why your own bed is paradise after being discharged from the hospital.

6

I pulled myself from a deep, hollow place. An air of warmth embraced me, even though the hospital smells and clatter on tile were still there, just beyond my curtained barrier.

I glanced at my wife. Her legs curled under, and her face was patterned by the rough cloth of a folding chair. She stared vacantly in the direction of a collapsing saline bag, dripping through tubes into a taped-over vein on a patient to my left. She was lost in another zone—a place I'd just visited and had barely returned from.

Diana had that tight-lipped, raised-forehead expression as if she was waiting for an unknown answer. I could see questions rotating behind her eyes. *Is he okay? How bad is it? Am I going to be a young widow? What are the chances? Will this happen again?* There seemed to be a hundred more questions, traveling in an arc of destruction like machine gun fire—all of them just as deadly. The unanswered questions seemed to be breaking her *things-are-okay* façade like a herd of stampeding buffalo.

I was worried about her. She looked emotionally drained— wilted. She hadn't noticed that I had woken. I clutched at my heart then drifted back into exhaustion. My body floated away on a give-in-to-tiredness wave as I became aware once again of the hospital parade—the clanking wheels and the energetic aides pushing machines our way. My attitude tasted sour. My tongue lay limp, dry, and lifeless on the floor of my mouth. The evening crew was arriving.

A pretty blonde, three weeks beyond a much-needed bleach job, came bubbling in. All smiles and dimples, she pushed a tray of vials and chirped the obvious: "I'm here to draw some blood."

My eyes met hers, and I could feel that they were not much more than slits of annoyance. I had given enough blood to make Dracula undo a belt buckle. I thought about giving her a corny response along the lines of, *Well, where are your pencil and paper?* Instead, I rolled up the sleeve of my hospital gown and said, "Okay, you get one try."

She looked at my arm, tapped it a few times, and smiled. "With those veins, one try is all it should take."

I am thin for a heart patient—165 pounds—so my blue veins are like road maps and are clearly visible just under my skin. An overhead light twinkled above the south-facing curtain, and I came to life. Diana folded her chair up and stretched.

"You have just become my favorite blood-taking person but remember that the supply is limited." After a brief pause, I continued, "You know, I used to sell that stuff in college for pen and beer money."

"And, which did you buy more of?" the tech asked, with a smirk that brought out her dimples.

"You are quick. Actually, I received the pens from my mom."

She lacquered my veins with alcohol and inserted the needle with a steady, skillful poke. I grimaced but didn't need to. My blood rushed into a series of vials. The tech then ran a small gizmo over my blue wrist band; with hospitals working on balance sheets, I would be billed for this bloodletting within minutes. She labeled each vial with my name, patient number, and insurance information. My blood was packed and ready for the lab.

She stopped five feet away, turned around, and nodded her head toward the vials. "You know, I'm not paying you for this." Her eyes smiled deliberately. She smacked her lips with a light touch of fingertips. Her blonde hair flipped with a sudden jerk of her head. She turned and left.

I looked at Diana. "I guess I will be supplying the pen and beer money now if I can afford it after this."

Next, a balding technician pushed a portable x-ray machine into the room. The machine made jerky, quick movements and finally screeched to a stop after banging the IV stand and the corner of the Stryker hospital bed. The machine reminded me of a crane, though it was bulky and lacked the grace. The top bobbed in sporadic movements as the technician maneuvered the head of the metal bird over my chest. He wedged an uncomfortable square plate beneath my back, repositioning it several times to find the exact spot that produced barely tolerable pain for me. He pressed on my shoulders, making sure the x-ray plate was directly against my sore back. I grinned, as though I was enjoying all of it.

He put a protective vest over his blue shirt and asked my wife to step behind the machine for a moment so she wouldn't absorb the rays. I asked why the sick people weren't protected like the healthy people.

I gained little comfort from his reply: "It's just a small dose. Never enough to harm you."

"Then why is everyone else hiding behind barriers, as though grenades are being tossed?"

He ignored me as he exchanged one hard plate for another behind my back. He knew I was too sedated and ill to fight. I did know that if I was healthy, I would want to be behind a mechanical barrier with a lead vest, helmet, and safety goggles. The technician could stand in front of me, deflecting or absorbing any particles that made it through the barrier. I made a mental note to be healthy the next time I entered a hospital. Good advice.

"This is so we can know the situation," the tech mumbled absently, even though I hadn't asked.

After a lot of clanking, gliding, humming noises, the machine folded itself up and the tech drove it away, Diana was back, holding my hand. *She must actually love me, to hold a such a sweaty and clammy palm.* I told her I felt much better now that I had lain on a stiff, square plate and been bombarded with invisible particles everyone else was hiding from.

Diana assured me with a soft scolding. "You're going to be fine."

"Am I a different color? I feel as though I should be glowing florescent green or have patchy, purple blotches on my skin." I glanced around for a mirror, with no luck. "Be straight with me—what color am I?" I proceeded to turn my arms, rotating from the elbow, as though looking for color changes. I held them out to her for inspection.

"Don't worry," Diana said. "Once you take a shower, I'm sure it will wash right off. If it doesn't, I'm sure we can find shirts that match."

"Real funny. No, I mean it! What color? I feel very different." I held one leg out, shaking it, imitating a seizure. My tongue lopped from one side of my mouth.

It was certainly a bit of much-needed fun, but I found that playing used up too much energy. I inhaled deeply to alleviate the dizziness. My stupid heart couldn't even take joking around without kicking me into a hole.

Taking a deep breath, Diana responded sarcastically, "You are the color of absurdity, and you wear it well."

Then she leaned down, kissing my forehead, and whispered, "You doing okay?"

"I'd rather have an éclair."

Her soft voice rose an octave in volume as she backed away from my forehead. "They said you couldn't even have a drink of water. I'm no physician, but I assume an éclair is out of the question." She rubbed her soft chin. "They called it *NPO* and said you could have nothing by mouth. Shouldn't it be *NBM*?" Diana shook her head. "Whatever. Just relax and don't think about food."

"As long as they don't make me lie on that garden brick again."

The soft voice came close to my ear again, with the inflection of a smile. "You're silly!"

"That's what draining me of all those vials of blood does. That and lying on this stupid bed in a building full of sick people."

I was losing energy again and fading. "A heart attack is a silly thing," I slurred. I began falling into the type of sleep where you hear voices and movement around you but resist answering or moving. The strength just wasn't there. The exterior whisperings quit making sense. I tumbled down the path to dreamland—and its blank screen.

Later, my wife told me I slept a full thirty-five minutes before the next round of machines, techs, and nurses rumbled in. Thank God for other patients! It was a busy day in the ER. I welcomed other people getting attention—or abuse, depending on your point of view. *Others are sick, too. Bother them. Test them. Drain their fluids. Let me have my moment of peace.*

The x-ray tech had left the curtain partially open, and I could *see* other patients instead of just hearing their groans and cries. I began noticing real people—people with expressions of concern or fright or indifference. We were all under the spell of being ill and violated. We had all been somewhat whole before arriving here, but something had happened to each one of us to deprive us of that. We ended up here, with privacy guarded by no more than a fluttering curtain and with arms attached to tubes and needles. Yesterday was better for all of us. Yesterday, we saw basketball game, or drove children to dance lessons or had ice cream cones. Today, we're all here, health insurance cards in hand. If we had the choice, I assume we would all go back to yesterday.

It occurred to me that the insurance industry would prefer yesterday as well. Their charts were changing and premiums expanding as more of us crowded for our places in the ER. They sat back in those tall glass buildings with giant acronyms displaying their name, pulling their hair out as they worried about their own bottom line. The stockholders were grumbling. Computers were clicking out of control. Secretaries wanted more days off, and salespeople demanded better commissions. And here we were, restless, waiting for expensive tests and overpriced rooms.

I perused the ER, my neck stabilized by an abundance of pillows built of collapsed air and little stuffing. *Almost-pillows*, I would call them. If you bunched five together, perhaps a real pillow would emerge. I looked out at the other people in my section of the ER. Their complacent, worried faces glanced back, then quickly turned away so I wouldn't know they were looking. I did the same.

The fear in the air was so thick you could scoop it up in a cupped hand. Fear darkened eyes and brought tears that couldn't be wiped away. It quivered slowly down spines. It thickened breathing and held fast. It was the binding we all shared. It was the thing we could all have done without.

Across from my space, a husky girl of about eighteen reclined in her bed; there was blood on her arm and the front of her blouse. She was crying in spurts, her head rocking back and forth. A man in a Raider's t-shirt held her good arm and rubbed the top of her head as it swayed. The eyes of fear and pain glanced at me without focus. Earlier I had overheard the words *compound fracture*, and looking at her now, I decided they must have been referring to her. A young doctor was cleaning her wounds with large Q-tips and a plastic bowl of a lime-green solution. Not a color I would associate with sterility. I would think of blue or maybe light purple—but maybe that's because those are colors of the popsicles I enjoy. It was hard to separate the two.

Next to me, I could see age-spotted feet and a gray-haired head of an older man. The curtain obscured my view of the rest of him. The toes curled inward with untrimmed nails, infested with yellowish fungus. A full head of hair escaped outward from the other end, looking like Einstein's, only shorter. I could hear a grumbling sound as he labored to breathe. His chin was dotted with salt-and-pepper stubble. His eyebrows were bushy and matched his apparent disregard for the hair on top of his head. A comb would have stopped dead in the tangle.

A concerned woman with him told him repeatedly that his glasses were on the dresser at home. It was easy to speculate about what brought him here without all the facts. Based on his slurred speech, I suspected he was suffering from Alzheimer's or drunkenness or a stroke. Or maybe he was just trying to drive his wife of many years completely crazy. But what did I know? I was basing my entire diagnosis on skinny ankles and a gray-haired raisin of a head.

Two curtains to my right sat a female patient, enveloping a low ER bed. She appeared soft and fragile and was having a difficult time situating her large body. Her cheeks were puffy and splattered with deep-pink blotches. Her eyes were sunken and black. Her body had been expanded by fries, burgers, and cokes—or maybe by bad heredity. Her mouth hung open, as though she were a young, chubby bird waiting for a worm to be dropped in. Perspiration glimmered on her face, neck, and arms.

A single tear circled her cheek and dropped from her chin onto white linen. She caught me looking at her and gave me the most radiant, good-natured smile I had seen in a long time. I didn't look away. I smiled back, raising my hand in a gesture that said *hello*. She returned my signal. I was worried about her. Without words, we became friends.

Her husband—or perhaps an older brother—stood at her side. The man either shared her genetics or had sat at the same abundant table. He looked disinterested, impatient, and inconvenienced by having to wait there. I felt bad for her as I watched his scowl, one that appeared far too practiced. Finally, a nurse approached with a blood pressure cuff and words of concern. My new hospital friend looked up with an expression of relieved expectation just as the drape closed.

There were two other patients in the room, each with closed drapes. I could hear mumblings and coughing, but no discernible words. There were no free beds that I could see. It appeared to be a time of feast, not famine, for the medical profession.

Nurses, doctors, and technicians streamed quickly in and out of the curtained-off areas. It was a fast-paced work environment. Most of the staff were concerned and kind. Some wore faces of arrogance and duty. Some smiled with a glance as they passed me. Others had tunnel vision down to a science. Some walked with happy strides. Others took each deliberate step as though squishing overgrown bugs on the tiled floor. It was all very amusing to watch. But then, I am easily entertained, especially when medicated and peeing orange.

7

A nurse came through the ER doors with a whoosh, eyes
intent on me. She pushed an off-white, square machine centered
on a stainless-steel table; the wheels squealed like mice. It was
clearly a machine built for medical utility—very plain, with
connector holes and switches. I had previously seen this same
nurse visiting other patients, IV bottles in hand. I recognized her
look of authority and her purposeful gait.

The nurse assumed an athletic stance as she and the cart
stopped at my side. Careless shaving had left patches of spotted
neglect on her muscular legs. Her thick, curly hair was pulled
back over her ears, held in place by a wooden butterfly clip
before it billowed out midway down her back. Her face was
happy, but she wasn't smiling. Her name tag said *Elaine
Anderton, R.N.*

Nurse Elaine introduced herself and the machine, a formality
I found amusing. She said it was an electrocardiograph that
would measure the electrical impulses of my heart and let the
doctor know more about how my heart was doing after the
cardiac arrest.

During college, I had worked in a hospital operating room, so
I had a basic grasp of what the electrocardiograph did. It
recorded valleys and peaks of heart impulses. It produced
specific spikes for the upper chamber of the heart and others for
the lower chamber. There was a short, straight line; a rest period;
then a duplicate of the original spikes. Important fact: If the
machine showed some version of that, you were alive.

From the day I learned of my cardiac arrest, I had a favorite
pump in my life. Some people have favorite cars and prized cats.
I have a favorite pump. I barely knew it existed prior to my time
in the Emergency Room; in fact, I'm sure I never even gave a
passing thought to my pump's twenty-four/seven ability. But

suddenly, the working coronary system was extremely important to me. Funny how only a few days earlier, toast and jam were so important to me.

Nurse Elaine explained it would only take a short time for her to run the test. Then she told me the ER had two of these machines, almost as if she expected me to sit up and applaud. The machine looked like the back of my stereo amplifier. The term *wired for sound* kept pinging around in my head.

I was dry-shaved in the spots on my chest that Nurse Elaine deemed necessary; I quickly noticed there was no pattern or artistic intent. I'm not exactly simian, but I do have a thicket of chest hair, though translucent blonde. My skin stung slightly where her razor cut in haphazard patches. *When this adventure is over,* I thought, *I am going to look absurd. The neighbors will talk. Gossip will flow. There will be torches and pitchforks in our front yard. Or maybe I'll just keep my shirt on.*

Nurse Elaine attached little foam squares with snaps in the center on what appeared to be random parts of my chest and sides where I had been shaved. Then she attached one on my ankle, just for good measure—or maybe in case I tried to get away. She quickly and methodically clipped color-coded electrodes to each snap.

Nurse Elaine then flipped a switch, verifying everything was in order. The machine purred. After looking at the printout, Nurse Elaine seemed content, as though it made perfect sense. With a rub of her chin and without any fanfare, she said, "That's it," unhooked the clips, disconnected the wires, wrapped everything up, and put it all away in a metal box attached to the machine. She was so efficient that she was gone before I realized it.

I had periodically felt a little closer to the other side since having my heart attack. Without the doctor reading my printout, I knew that my spikes were not perfect. I could sense murmurings in my chest. There were definite off-beat moments. It was like a melodrama in my chest as my heart sped up and produced extra, unexpected beats. I'm not saying this heart attack stuff wasn't fascinating; I'm just saying it involved high anxiety involved. The whole time my mood flowed like liquid, washing back and forth between enjoying all the attention to sensing the threatening doom of reality.

Humor was my release. I joked with the nurses and technicians, "Is there a discount if I draw my own blood? Could I get music instead of all these beeps from my monitor? It would be so much more soothing."

And I could still jest with my wife. "You can go back to work if you want. I'll call when they're done."

I used the humor to insulate myself from the absoluteness of death. If I could joke and laugh, I must not be too sick. However, I was finding that humor was suddenly much more difficult. The obstacles seemed greater. It did help when the staff responded with grins and reciprocal sarcasm. I breathed in their happy spirit. It gave me a momentary flight from the phrases *heart attack* and *cardiac arrest*.

I play a similar game with clothes. If I wake with an upset stomach, a backache, a hangover, or sore muscles following excessive exercise, I dress better. I shower and shave to excess and brush my teeth twice. I put on my most respectable pants, a perfectly ironed shirt, highly polished shoes, and a flamboyant matching tie. In other words, I feel like crap, but the décor looks great. It's my way of fooling my body into feeling better. And it works. I have made it through many a miserable day by enjoying positive comments and walking upright when I know I should be in bed moaning into a pillow. Instead, I suffer less and save my sick days for times when I'm healthy enough to enjoy waterskiing behind a boat or fishing a clear creek. It works for me.

Don't get me wrong. I don't think my hospitalization would have been better had I been wearing a three-piece suit while perched on the gurney. I couldn't have fooled even myself. My frightened eyes and discolored complexion would have given away my issues long before anyone had a chance to notice the three-piece suit. But I would have been the best-dressed patient in the ER.

My thoughts kept me amused. I lay there in an open-backed, slipped-over-the-head dress they call a hospital gown. I always thought a gown was a woman's formal dress. If my mom wore *this* gown out on the town with my dad, I'd wonder what kind of affair she was attending. I was already scarred for life from watching certain patients walk back and forth to the bathroom. I'd had enough glimpses of body crevices and fat folds to cause night terrors for years to come. The ill apparently have no modesty and little self-respect. I understand their situation. Once pain and suffering reach a certain level, it's hard to care.

As it was, my ER time was spent gasping for air, making sarcastic comments, trying not to watch exposed patients, and feeling the quick, offshoot spasms called angina. It was to be the beginning of an interesting sequence of days—a situation that would ultimately last for years.

Thoughts of my son Kyle slammed into my mind. I grabbed Diana's hand, and I wasn't gentle. *I need to be healthy for Kyle. He has enough problems. What a time for my heart to go wonky.* I felt my eyes water up.

"Kyle?" I asked.

Her face slackened. "He's at Nate's house. I had them pick him up after school."

"And Tim?" My son Jeremy was in Oregon for work and Jim was in the Marines at Camp Lejeune, North Carolina.

"I called Patti. She's aware we won't be picking them up tonight. She'll let them know later when we know more about your condition."

Patti was my children's mother, and they lived with her most of the time. Though Patti and I were no longer married, we had a congenial friendship that always considered what was best for our boys—Jim, Jeremy, and Tim.

"My condition's easy. I've got a stupid heart, that has stupid beats, that's put me in this stupid hospital."

"Enough with the stupid." Diana laughed.

I cracked up. My arm yanked against the inserted IV and tape; I winced and felt another jolt of pain rip through my chest and down to my calves. I straightened and pressed against the raised gurney, taking in soft breaths and waiting for my muscles to relax. Diana stroked my forehead. Her mouth hung open as if she wanted to say something.

"You okay?" she whispered.

I waited a few moments for the last strain of agony to melt. My eyes narrowed as I panned over my IV and heart monitor cables cuddled like newborn snakes twisting around my upper body. Despair drained through my body for a few minutes. I sucked in a slow, deep breath.

My eyes stared at the floor. "Kyle. Does he have any appointments today?"

"Nothing for about a week." Diana stretched her neck, then she stared at the ceiling for a moment. "Then he's scheduled for radiation at Primary Children's Hospital."

"I really don't have time for this coronary crap right now."

Diana patted my hand. "It'll be okay."

I was happy to see the next machine heading my way to probe my slothful heart. It arrived with little celebration. It came with a lumpy, short girl whose bangs were sprayed stiff and combed to resemble a black-iron gate on her forehead.

She was all business. She had on one of those hospital-blue tops festooned with tiny, dancing figures of Mickey Mouse and Goofy, holding hands. The gaiety stopped there. Her black hair was pulled back from those bangs into a ponytail that drifted down a hunched back. Her white sneakers squeaked on the tile as she dragged the sides of her wide feet. They didn't seem to be chained and weighted, but she moved as though they were. *Quasimodo to cardio, Quasimodo to cardio,* I heard over my mind's loudspeaker.

Her mouth was a straight line under a thin nose that didn't fit her bulbous cheeks and lava-layered neck. She spoke very precisely. Her bottom lip never moved, similar to a ventriloquist or a cowboy with Skoal tucked between his cheek and gum. Sound came from her mouth without any visual clues. "I'm going to take a picture of your heart," she said.

I looked up at her seriously. "That sounds wonderful! How much for two four-by-fives and one eight-by-ten? And could we bunch all the gurneys together and get kind of a family portrait?"

My wife bit her lip. A smile edged up on one side. Her eyes squinted. It wasn't all that funny, but it must have really resonated with Diana. I know I needed the lighter mood.

The nurse's eyes bored through me. Her lips moved this time, emphatically, with "Sir" thrown at me like an expletive, as well as every word thereafter: "these . . . are . . . not . . . those . . . kind . . . of . . . pictures."

"Oh, so they're video?" I tried, turning on the charm.

"Yes, they are like a short video of your heart pumping," she said.

"VHS or DVD? I could use either."

She glanced at my wife for help, then looked toward the door as if searching for a way out.

My wife tried to appease her. "Don't listen to him; just do what you have to do. He's on medication! The sicker he is, the more his mouth moves." As she spoke, Diana held her cupped hands out, tapping her thumbs together like two fighting adversaries. She smiled, giving me a scrunched-eye look. Her idea of an evil glare was pathetic.

"Oh, yeah, make fun of the invalid," I quipped, my arms folded on my belly in defense.

Diana opened and closed her fingers against the thumb imitating a puppet yapping at me. After a brief period of silence, she said, "You forget, I've been around you with the flu—and other times with your prattling ailments."

I ignored her and turned to the nurse tech. "So, getting a copy is out of the question?"

I was fully ignored by the pudgy, non-emotional nurse. She looked everywhere but at me. I stared intently at her eyes. She could feel it. She tried hard to keep busy, preparing the echocardiograph. I began to feel bad, emotionally and physically. My body was wearing down again. Plus, I think I scared her. Humor works for me, but not everyone. Especially when they (anyone other than me) are on the receiving end of it. Oh, what the hell. I was having fun with this heart attack. It was the last one I planned to have.

As Nurse Quasimodo put the wet, semi-liquid, conductor gel on my chest that enabled the machine to take clearer pictures, I was slowing down significantly. I was still gray and fully horizontal, but I had no witty humor. Wow, I was losing ground.

It felt like success to just take a breath fourteen times a minute. My body was struggling, and I feared I had no reserve energy.

I closed my eyes and became somewhat incoherent. There was some labor involved, which I had no strength for. I was in that state of almost sleep, where you can hear the voices, maybe even make out certain words, but you are drifting away from them. I knew the point of being pulled down, deep, but having no awareness or recollection of actual sleep. This seemed to be a habit now.

I don't know how long I was out. I'm sure the nurse was relieved. No more absurd questions from her patient. I was half asleep and probably still mumbling. Illness and fear blossoms with a terrible personality at times.

Time passed between heavy eyelids, annoying chatter, and boredom. Diana was locked into cell phone mode. Those things are so useful, and at the same time they are so annoying. Someday we will all have cell phones surgically implanted. We will blink hard and twitch several times to dial out. There will be groups of young girls and boys, all contorting their faces, dialing as they traverse the new stores and food courts in open malls across the country. Twitching will be rampant and commonplace. We will see it on Wall Street and at McDonalds, at Gold's Gym and at quick marts. Families will sit down to eat dinner and facially twitch to dial other people sitting down at the dinner table in other homes across the nation and the world. Dinner chatter will involve someone miles away. "Twitching like Rabbits" will be the slogan at Verizon Wireless, if they still exist. I envision a paradigm shift in communication with the implantable cell phone business. It will be like the change from mailing letters with actual stamps to e-mail.

But, for now, my wife had taken over the informational part of my emergency room experience, via cell phone. The data readings from the ER beeped and gurgled as the electronic machines prattled on. Nurses strolled through using terms like *stable* and *quietly resting* and one of the big ones—*waiting for the test results*.

I woke slowly from a deep medication- and pain-induced sleep. I sporadically heard fragments of a one-way conversation between my wife and an unknown caller. It was more like a briefing. "This is what *we* think is happening, based on the facts *we* have at this time."

I tried to raise my head toward the phone voice. Dizziness abated that abruptly. Diana leaned in front of me, giving hand signals and mouthing silent words I couldn't understand. She smiled and nodded, as if she knew I fully comprehended. I smiled back, as though it all made perfect sense. In her mind, a light bulb had gone on above my head. In my mind, it was a question mark, lit and flashing.

I have never been so complacent and pliable in such a frantic environment—or in any environment, for that matter. I was neither comfortable nor uncomfortable. I was on the edge of awakening but without full awareness or wonder. The scene in front of me just happened. My mind was held in a state of Vaseline, trying to be a solid, but oozing out on the fringes.

My cardiologist headed toward my chart. I hadn't realized I even had a chart. Should I worry? His eyebrows were pulled tightly enough to produce a migraine. Uh oh.

8

My chest tightened as I stared into the serious eyes of my cardiologist.

"How are you feeling right now?" Dr. Vandoven asked.

I was on one of those short-lived moments of vitality that I knew wouldn't last. With a hard, low-lung inhale, I said, "I'm feeling much better. But I'm like a boat with water in the carburetor, sucking air with a gargling sound. I don't think I'm running right." I waited for his response.

He switched posture, shifting weight from one side to the other. "No, you're not running right. But we are working on helping you through that as quickly as possible."

He paused and rubbed his chin. "All your labs are back. I have good news and bad news. The good news is that it's not what we initially feared." Initially, he explained, preliminary test results and my symptoms indicated an infected heart valve. "That would have required the leaping step of a heart transplant, which is associated with a high mortality rate."

This backache is getting worse by the second. A rush of fear shot adrenaline through my body, and every muscle seemed tied in knots around creaking bones. *This is the good news? Or was this his method of shock therapy?*

He went on. "But here's the bad news. Jef, you had a cardiac arrest, probably on Tuesday or Wednesday. I'm sure you knew that. Also, you have pericarditis, which is an inflammation of the pericardium, or the sack enclosing the heart."

Crap. So, I'm too young for this to happen—but it happened. Isn't the cardiac arrest bad enough? And now my pericardium, something I didn't even know I had, is swollen like a bloated pig.

Dr. Vandoven went on. "Pericarditis is present in 10 percent of heart cases, but usually people have it before having a heart attack. In contrast, yours apparently developed after the heart attack." He went on to say I would receive antibiotics for the pericarditis and that they would do additional tests to determine the extent of damage to my heart, probably an angiogram in the morning. His nurse had apparently scheduled that. He explained further that my heart had also swollen.

Crap. I even had this pericarditis backwards. I gazed at my chest with all the pads and wires attached. I envisioned my heart all misshapen and as big as a watermelon, quivering inside a giant leather sack.

To me, none of this sounded any better than the infected heart valve. It was more like, *Here is the bad news, and here is the other bad news*. The good news is your property is covered with twisted trees and metal debris, and the bad news is your house was tossed several miles during the tornado. *Wow! I am so relieved.*

"Is . . . that . . . bad?" Diana forced out.

"At this point, we are looking at all of the options," the doctor said. "We are admitting you to the hospital for a few days of observation. I have scheduled an angiogram tomorrow, and we will determine where we go from there." He went on to explain some things about my chemistry that I didn't comprehend. There was something about high bilirubin and low something else. I had no clue what bilirubin was, but I could tell from his voice that I didn't want it high.

"So, this is not a 'take-two-aspirins-and-call-me-in-the-morning' kind of thing?" I asked.

"Hardly. But with the medication, you should be feeling better in a few days. Do you want to know anything about the angiogram?"

I nodded weakly. *I want to know what the heck it is. I want to know that it's not painful. I want to know how it will make me feel better. I want to know anything else that I should know about it.*

He took a lot of time explaining and answering my questions. He drew diagrams of the heart and of the human body. Although he will never make a living at art, the drawings and arrows made me feel better. He explained the risks involved and the possible outcomes.

My mind swirled in a stew of diagnoses and outcomes. It was like two buddies planning a night on the town. I was more relaxed when our conversation ended—mostly because it ended. And man, was I hungry!

"Food and water! I need food and water." After the information overload, hunger hit quickly and seemed to spread from the top down. I was dizzy and my belly was making gurgling sounds. I am one of those people who must eat three times a day at specific intervals, or I get dizzy and cranky. My sister tells me I'm hypoglycemic. I think I just burn off food quickly.

"Yes, you can eat now," Dr. Vandoven said. "I will have the nurse order you something right away. They will take you to Room 204 in a few minutes. Your food tray will be there. I will check on you again before I leave tonight. Any questions?"

"Thousands, but I think I need to let this day's adventure simmer for a while. I'll ask some later, if it's all right."

He patted me on the shoulder and headed for the open door. He seemed to be big with the pat on the shoulder. It was comforting. His last statement was, "Rest. This is serious."

Diana followed him, catching him just outside the door. I could see her going into lawyer *voir dire* questioning mode. She is a glutton for answers. If she were at home, she would be locked onto all sorts of medical websites about the heart. She wants to know it all. Within a day or so, I knew she would have information, summaries, and notes on the latest studies, and she would have talked to doctors all around the country to learn the latest options for solving my cardiac problems. I knew terms like *pericarditis* and *cardiac infarction* would roll off her tongue.

Me? I'll settle for a meal and the basic truth about my condition. I don't care about herbal remedies, acupuncture treatments, how someone treats a heart attack in Peru, what minerals might do, which vitamins I might need, or the latest massage therapy for heart patients. I will change doctors if I don't feel good about one as a healer, but I'll put my full trust in one that has a conscience and is caring. Right then, I felt really good about my cardiologist.

About an hour and a half later, an orderly in regular blues came and wheeled me out of the emergency room. My body and mind were too worn to care about what they were doing to me. The hunger had vanished as if my cells were cannibalizing themselves. I was sedated, both pharmaceutically and naturally. I was ready for them to wheel me to whatever-the-hell floor they deemed necessary. I had been through days of horrid torture since my heart attack. I was headed to a room where they had food—or at least, the promise of food. *A burger and fries sound good, but I'm pretty sure it's not on the cardiac patient menu. I wonder how their sashimi is here? Or their veal piccata? What do cardiac care patients eat? I hoped it's not something off the Campbell's aisle.*

I considered my condition. Where was that high-octane, get-everything-done person? Where was that planning, constructing, thinking, working-on-five-projects-at-a-time human I used to be? I was the achiever formerly known as Jef. My mind was foggy. My body was tired. My back hurt. I looked like me, only a gray and weak version of me. My body felt somewhat familiar, but my insides felt like they were being pulled down by gravity from another planet. One minute my mind was sharp and humming quickly; the next, I was barely able to remember my name. *Get up . . . get up and do something. Anything. Go to work. Be better.* But the body that was formerly Jef listened to my thoughts of *do this* and *try that*, and my body simply ignored them.

I assumed some of my lost capability was related to the drugs I was taking. Some was also from the physical and personal shock of my heart attack and the fact that I hadn't gotten rapid treatment. And some was due to relying on doctors, RNs, LPNs, techs, and of course my loving wife to do everything for me. The last part was kind of nice. I wouldn't want to rely on others for too long, but right then I needed it. I was enjoying being a little pampered.

The orderly wheeled me into the elevator, and the doors clamped shut. The orderly glared at me as if deciding whether to take me to Room 204 or downstairs to the morgue. His look didn't raise my spirits. Diana held my hand in a solid grip. Was she making sure I had a pulse, or was she being caring? Those thoughts didn't help, either.

I had gotten used to my rather impaired hearing. There were several reasons for it. During my late teens, I had blown out the cilia in my ears while working at a loud discotheque at night and standing close to speakers the size of Ford Expedition. The tiny hairs deep in my ears that vibrate in response to outside sounds were exhausted. I envisioned them as limp, oversaturated angel hair spaghetti. But that wasn't all: add years of sixties rock and roll in my mother's basement, with me dancing, smiling, and swaying to the impossibly loud music. Later, people thought I didn't pay attention, never realizing that my ears barely worked.

But for some bizarre reason, my hearing had gotten better during the hours I had spent the hospital. I'm not sure why, but I knew *something* had happened. It sounded like the volume of the world had been cranked up, and vibrations flowed easily through the sterile hospital air. I could pick out a specific wheel of a gurney on the tiled floor. I imagined, by the sound, it had two small chunks of rubber missing, spaced an inch apart. I could tell when it crossed the color-coded, directional lines. The gurney could almost say, "This way to x-ray," or, "That way to the waiting room."

I heard smoker's laughter cackling through the air beyond the next room. I could hear the shuffle of feet in a nervous pattern on the tile—*pah dum, pah dum, pah dum,* the dance of anxiety. I listened as an air suction hose worked on someone's throat, and I heard the gagging response.

With my improved hearing, I differentiated between the way people walked. Some steps were slow, with a gliding motion. Others sounded quick and impatient as they hurried back and forth. There was one nurse who paced in a determined, cat-like way, and another who sounded like a drumbeat.

I am not sure if my hearing was radically better or if my concentration had increased. Did physiology change the ear canal, cilia, and tiny bones after a heart attack? I doubted it. I sought other options. Perhaps my ears had grown bigger? I looked for a mirror.

"Honey, are my ears growing?"

Diana put her cell phone down. "Yeah, they are enormous. How did you know?"

"I'm hearing things I haven't heard before."

She looked pleased. "Oh, that would be nice." Then sarcasm permeated her voice. "You mean you may be able to actually hear me?"

"No, not you specifically, just subtle things, like bugs and a light breeze."

"You've taken away my dream."

"Maybe your voice is the reason I can't hear you. You sound like Minnie Mouse. Try talking a little deeper, with a southern accent."

I felt a slight twist on my ear.

"Can you hear that?" Her voice was as forceful as her fingers.

"Loud and clear," I whined. "Remember, I'm ill. If you don't stop, I'll call that big nurse over there."

Diana smiled and took a breath. "I think I could take her."

"You know, I'm hearing you a lot better right now."

Diana smirked and slowly nodded her approval before she let go of my ear.

Dr. Vandoven woke me from a semi-conscious state. "Jef . . . Jef?" His voice blew the fog back. He gently squeezed my shoulder while Diana gripped my right hand. Twisting my neck from side to side, shaking my head, and blinking my blurry eyes, I was renewed.

"Sorry, I keep falling asleep." My voice echoed through my newly receptive ears.

"You're supposed to," the doctor said.

"Splendid, then I must be doing everything I should." My tongue darted around my mouth; instant disgust was painted on my lips from my arid, rancid-tasting breath.

It felt as if twenty-something hours had passed since I got to the hospital. A glance at the clock, though, revealed I had entered the ER only five hours earlier. With my internal clock set to hospital time, confusion rolled through my mind.

In the *real* world, the one without IV drips and blood draws, my hunger peaks as soon as I wake up, usually around seven; it hits again at eleven-thirty in the morning; then hunger strikes my internal clock at six for dinner. During the day, I can typically gauge time to within a few minutes by how my stomach feels. If I awaken at night, I have some internal time-tracking sense that lets me know within an hour or so of the exact time.

That doesn't happen in the hospital. As a patient, it's hard to tell whether you have endured a few minutes, an hour, or several days. Patients define time by nurse visits and medical tests. I've decided when one is ill, hunger doesn't play a big role. There is no breakfast time or lunch time or dinner time.

I learned how irrelevant time is in a hospital bed. I might know that I had two nurse visits, an x-ray, and a tray filled with pale-colored, gelatin-like stuff, with spurts of sleeping in between. But it's hard to know the real time, especially when they woke me for a check of vital signs every hour. And just when I thought I understand the shift changes, a nurse pulled a double, and was confused and out of luck again. If it hadn't been for the window in the room, I couldn't have told day from night. I probably doesn't matter much, because projects and work responsibilities are put on hold, but at the time it's totally disconcerting.

9

A calm, pleasant feeling settled in my chest as I looked quietly around my hospital room. There was rhythm to the intake of air in my lungs. The constant beeps and red lights of machines, the shuffling shoes against the hallway floor, and the blood pressure cuff filling and deflating became music. The sounds from outside my room—low-level gibberish and the clicking of high heels—added to the ambiance. Business as usual was going on all around me while I felt forever exhausted.

My wife sat in a corner chair, lazily reading. One eye loomed above the cover, peeping at me in two-minute intervals. Her legs were elevated on a folding chair, and her overall position was a chiropractor's dream of visits to come. Her hair was disheveled from a restless night. Yesterday's clothes showed signs of needing an iron—or, better still, a toss. Two small, empty milk cartons, one on its side, and a Kit Kat wrapper told me she'd eaten late (though not well).

The windows framed a display of gray-blue sky and quietly moving cirrus clouds. Flecks of dust sparkled in the light, moving in organized chaos. I took a strong breath and blew it out straight at the specks. To my delight, several seconds later they responded, twirling and dancing through the air. I regained a small amount of self-assurance. My manhood had returned—I could move dust.

My body was immobile, my eyes watching everything in couldn't-care-less motions. A plastic, puke-yellow pitcher and a Styrofoam cup with a straw sat on a rolling gray table. I lay on sheets and a pillow, all smelling of antiseptic wash.

Inactivity settled on me in a welcoming way. I was unconcerned. My breathing was steady and, according to one machine, I was receiving 97 percent oxygen. The plastic prongs in my nose assuredly had something to do with that.

My stomach told my brain I was hungry. My brain was too sedated and exhausted to care.

Whenever there is calm, the opposite follows—and it was no different for me. Suddenly there was a knock followed by the clanging of a food tray against the solid wood door. There seemed to be a bit of a scuffle between the tray and the door, and the door seemed to be winning. The persistence of the tray finally won out.

A lanky angel with carefully calibrated slop (I mean food) arrived with her imitation circus shoes, banging into all sorts of things as she scurried with my tray to the table. Her smiling lips seemed out of place. She came at me like a starfish, all arms and legs protruding from her center. The tray teetered in one unsteady hand. What I later found to be a next-day menu was held between the thumb and forefinger of her other hand. It all seemed so clumsy, careless, and entertaining. But I needed her simple silliness in a building of gray and doom. She was cute and cheerful.

"Oh, whoops!" she exclaimed, her smile vanishing as my Styrofoam cup unceremoniously emptied onto the industrial blue carpet.

I smiled reassuringly. Her name tag proclaimed her to be Lucy from Food Services.

"Mr. Huntsman?" she asked, her head tilted to one side. Her smile returned on high beam.

"Only . . . if you're Lucy," I answered.

The spill of my cup had brought my wife to attention. Diana's face cautioned me, her lips mouthing *Be nice*. While she didn't say a word, she pulled an imaginary zipper across her tightened lips.

"Uhh . . . yes, I am." Lucy was half-smiling but seemed to be slightly lost with a touch of anxiety. It was obvious the spill had thrown her off her normal game.

"Well, then, I must be Mr. Huntsman, but you can call me Jef. Okay?" I waited a few beats, adding, "How are you doing today?"

"Uhhh . . . fine?" she said as if there might be a rebuttal from me. She set the tray down carefully, taking two military steps away from the table. Like a light turning on, Lucy's smile came back to full beam. Her bubbling vitality came out. She looked from the spill to various places around the room. Her neck cranked and stretched. Her feet pivoted around the room in a concerned search mode.

"Good for you," I replied.

The tension in her eyes eased when she saw a stack of towels folded neatly on a shelf. She bounced over to them. First, she blotted, and then she vigorously rubbed the spill. Within a few moments, a satisfied grin formed dimples on her cheeks. Lucy tossed the bleached towels into a laundry basket a couple of feet away.

After she finished mopping the spill, Lucy stood and looked hesitantly at me without speaking, slowly rubbing both hands together. I assumed she was waiting to be excused, but I didn't let her off. I returned her smile. Her damp hands looked tight, and she released them only enough to interlock her fingers prayerfully. Her posture was at ease, but her face, neck, and arm muscles were taut in anticipation, the cartilage and blue veins poking out slightly.

"This must be the first course," I said. "Could you just keep them coming? And I could use a wine list."

Lucy stood still and bit her lip, an uneasy fear behind her smile. She pivoted slightly as though ready to flee. I don't think anyone had talked to her all day. Her eyes glanced over at Diana, who was back to reading her book. "Oh, you need water," she said as she turned to grab a cup.

"Lucy." I pointed with a white plastic fork. "What would you suggest to accompany this solid, mustard-looking stuff here?" I began poking it. My eyebrows rose for effect.

Lucy remained half twisted away. Her teeth were about to draw blood from her lips. Her smile was harder to make out. She glanced at the spill and the door and then to my tray.

Diana came to Lucy's rescue, tossing another towel on the floor to cover the darkened spot. "Now it's gone."

A small smile filled Lucy's face briefly, until she heard my voice again.

"What exactly *is* this?" I asked as I tried sticking my fork through something somewhat rectangular and camel colored.

Her lips released the words reluctantly. "Chicken. Uhhh, chicken, I think." Her head nodded in agreement with herself.

"Jef, just eat!" said Diana.

After a brief silence, Diana turned to Lucy. "Thank you for bringing the tray; he is starving." Without moving her head, her eyes turned to mine. "He's a touch delirious."

Lucy turned to leave. As she approached the door, the bounce returned to her feet.

Before she managed to get through the door, I held up the plastic fork again. "I guess a house white would be fine."

She turned to look at me, giving me that lost look again. "Uhhh . . . sir?"

Diana interrupted. "Lucy, thank you. Just go, you'll be better off."

I pointed my fork at Diana. "Are we, or are we not, here to get better and have a little fun?" I figured I'd get some respect with that fork.

Diana was emphatic. "No!"

"But—"

"Yes, get better. But have fun? Teasing the staff is not the definition of fun."

I understood. I dismissed my thoughts and focused on the tray, working on the things I recognized. The cookie and boxed juice were first.

As the hours and days progressed, Lucy and I became friends. She had a brother in the army (ours, I think), and a mother who did hair in her basement. She paid $52.50 to her mom for room and board. She explained the reason for the odd amount twice, but I still didn't get it. She took a short walk with her dog, a spaniel named Quickie, every night.

She had a quickie with Quickie every night. I like that.

Lucy's boyfriend was in jail for writing bad checks. According to her, he didn't mean to. He happened to find a checkbook lying on the asphalt in front of a Seven-Eleven. There were still five checks in it, and one thing led to another. She visited him on her days off.

Thinking back, my first night of EVER staying in a hospital was filled with anxiety that was laced with an odd, forced contentment. Sleep was sporadic. I tried to dismiss thoughts about my morning angiogram. The night nurse had said it would be nothing—but there is no such thing as "nothing" in a hospital. *Everything* is "something" in a medical facility. The procedure involved pushing a tube from my thigh to my heart in veins pulsing with life-giving blood, then releasing radioactive dye into those veins—and that didn't sound like "nothing" to me. It may be routine for hospital personnel, but it sounded completely intrusive from my point of view. *Maybe they'd let me try it on one of them first.*

I slept a bit and worried a lot. Diana stayed with me. Kyle was with his grandma and Tim was with his bio-mom.

The sun rose on a soft, silent morning. I stared out through the window; snow was falling so slowly and delicately it appeared to never hit the ground. Large, diaphanous flakes swung as if on strings, dipping lower with each pendulous movement. Diana was curled on a chair, clutching onto two hospital pillows as she slept soundly, her neck tilted at an angle begging for some Tylenol. It was uncomfortable to watch her contorted sleep. I looked back to the window and the snow.

Light made the flakes twinkle. My eyelids drooped as my body floated away.

Suddenly a full bladder hit me with urgency. A panic swept from my groin to my throat. I unsnapped wires and wound IV lines into a lasso, quietly and quickly, holding my breath between clamped lips. I ignored the nurse's button except to push it away from me and deep into the sheets.

I sat up on the edge of the bed; my head spun from sitting up too quickly. I gained equilibrium with steady breaths while twisting my legs like a rubber band. With urgent force I unsnapped the wires now yanking my chest. I flung them and the silly oxygen thing from my fingers. With my hospital sock-covered toes against the floor, I stood, grabbing the IV tree tightly with both hands, the transparent tubes dangling from above. I was wobbly as I walked carefully to the bathroom. An irritating beeping machine warned of my detachment from a monitor behind me. *Tattletale.*

I made it to the bathroom door just as the nurse came busting into my room. Diana woke up in sleepy, disoriented spurts. The nurse pointed her index finger at me, asking in an accusing tone of voice, "Where are you going?" I pointed to the bathroom. Her scowl made me want to raise my hands in surrender as though I was breaking and entering. *Someone called the nurse police. Foiled again.*

She scolded me. "You need to call us for help." She was babbling on about the perils and liability related to me taking seven whole steps to the bathroom.

I responded in the weak voice of someone who had been caught. "You're going to help me urinate?"

"No! We need to make sure you are walking okay. We don't want you slipping and falling. Things light up at the desk if your monitor plugs are disconnected. We think you're having a heart attack."

Two more nurses came in to see if I was well enough to pee. My audience was expanding. The other nurses looked at me with expressions like the first. *I was a naughty boy.* My good-patient status was shrinking with every tight-faced look I received.

Diana broke in. "Why didn't you wake me?"

Wow! *Everybody* wanted to help me pee. I had really broken the rules by trying to urinate by myself.

I asked as contritely as possible, "May I use the bathroom now? There's a lot of pressure in my bladder." I was holding my legs tightly together.

"Sure, go ahead," said the first female nurse with an approving, yet skeptical, nod. Her voice had a slight baby-talk tone to it. "But leave the door slightly open."

The other nurses nodded in unison. My wife gave an underhanded gesture of fingers and wrist, signaling me to go. I smiled in relief and pushed the metal IV stand in front of me as I entered whatever privacy a semi-closed door would give.

I said, "Thank you," as though I should be happy about their permission. *I am not a five-year-old. My type A personality is having a hard time with this level of control.* I had heart failure. I peed, mumbling expletives to myself.

I glanced down. My urine was not orange. *Oh, happy day.*

Washing my hands was difficult with tiny tubes taped to my wrist and with hair pulling tape inside my elbows from previous bloodletting. I dried off with six-inch brown squares of paper. I was annoyed and I was lightheaded.

I exited the washroom, finding my wife and the morning nurse hovering in wait to prepare me for naptime. I was relieved they weren't holding graham crackers and milk or handing me a blankie.

Just as I made it into bed, a gurney slammed into the door frame as a young orderly came storming in to retrieve me for my angiogram. He was just peeping into his twenties, with the pimples of a teen dotting his cheeks. His hair was wet and combed. An attempt had been made at maturity by the thirty-seven hairs sprouting from his extended, narrow chin. He wore blue scrubs and a crucifix on a dull, silver chain. His index and middle finger were stained amber from smoking.

A deep voice boomed from him, as if through a loudspeaker, unfitting for his small mouth. It was the voice of a sports announcer. He may have looked weak, but he firmly imparted authority. "Are you Jef Huntsman? I'm here to take you to the cath lab."

I nodded my head as he checked my wristband to see if I was lying. Right: I'm going to take someone else's place to have a tube shoved through my veins from my groin to my heart. *Mmmm, maybe I should have considered getting someone to take my place.*

There are very few situations more humiliating than a gurney ride. You are wheeled around and set on display as you pass lights, ceiling tiles, and gawking eyes while you wonder if you're going to die. It's the same thing that happens on the freeway at an accident—people slow as they search for blood and gore. Diana and the staff nurse studied me, trying to be nonchalant as we entered the elevator. There was pity in their eyes. The dread of the day hit as the elevator dropped two floors and I was ping-ponged through the doors. Out into the florescent light again, I was once more on exhibit for the eyes of strangers. They stared unabashedly, and I could imagine the thoughts racing through their minds. *Where is he going? What happened? How bad is it? Is it contagious?*

At the double doors, Diana was dismissed. She gave me a kiss on my forehead, and I was wheeled away through several push-button-operated doors.

The operating room nurses greeted me, slid me onto the OR table, and busied themselves with duties they had clearly performed before. Dr. Vandoven came in, smiling, then patted me on the arm. He asked inconsequential questions while the nurses put new, white sheets over me and strapped my right arm to an extension board. My doctor patted me again, letting me know he'd be back shortly. One of the female nurses shaved half of my groin; any sense of modesty flew right out the door. One of the nurses wrapped two-inch tape around her fingers and patted it quickly around the shaved area to remove any excess shaved hair. *Ouch.* A sticky, clear patch was attached to my inner thigh.

The room was meat-locker cold. I began shivering. A saint of a nurse brought me a heated blanket as thin as cheesecloth. Removing the original, she covered me with the warm one and then with another warm blanket. The warm blankets were adjusted as a blue blanket was taken from a stainless-steel table and draped over me from chin to toe. A cutout hole allowed cold air on my exposed inner thigh.

Something they put in my IV flushed my face and relaxed me into unconsciousness.

Much later, I was half awake when Dr. Vandoven shared the results of the angiogram with me and Diana. He kept showing me an x-ray that looked like a shadowy night filled with white tree branches—not artsy enough for a frame, but it had a certain appeal. He mentioned bypass surgery, a lot of blockage, and that I would be released in a day or two so I could heal enough for surgery.

I began to hear my heart gurgling and sputtering. A lump as big and unreliable as a Ford Fiesta settled in my chest. I wasn't about to fall from my horse, but this news certainly hit me with the reality of death and taxes. I'd rather have the taxes.

One thing I was very proficient at in the hospital was sleep. My mind and body were overpowered with exhaustion. Even awake, I was always on the verge of napping. Friends and family stopped by to visit, and I forced myself into a sedated alertness. I joked with them but fell asleep before they could respond. There was no offense intended—I was simply emotionally and physically depleted. I could manage about fifteen minutes of conversation and then, without warning, I fell sound asleep in mid-sentence.

I was falling to sleep again when three short taps on the door warned me of incoming checkups. *Crap.*

The nurse arrived in silent sneakers. My mind blinked and tried to re-adjust the picture. She was different from the regular hospital staff. She was a little too pretty. I have never watched *General Hospital* (at least not that I would admit), but my new nurse was straight off the set. More of a model than a nurse, she had big, childlike eyes filled with a touch of concern; hair curled into soft ringlets; a petite nose; professional makeup; a body tailored by aerobic workouts; and the posture of a model on the runway. A hint of a grin came from pale, pink lipstick. Her long eyelashes fluttered, raising youthful wisdom lines on her lightly tanned forehead. Her six-foot frame moved with small, delicate steps to my bedside.

A warm Texas accent told me, "I'm your nurse for the next ten hours. Can I get you anything?"

"Tell me all about the Lone Star State."

"Jef!" warned Diana.

"No, oh no, I might have had too much pain medication. I seem to be feeling rather dizzy."

Diana interrupted. "Rather dizzy? *Rather?* I've never heard you use such a formal word before. If you're *rather* dizzy, perhaps you'd *rather* get some sleep."

"I use *rather* all the time."

"When? When do you use it all the time?"

"You know . . . like when I say, rather this, or rather that, or rather the other."

"Your nose is getting longer, Pinocchio."

"Yes, it rather is. Isn't it?"

The pretty nurse stood, patiently waiting for my wife and me to finish our banter. Her arms were crossed. It was clear she was becoming impatient and was trying to figure us out.

My pain-pill-blurred vision and my bobbing head looked toward the nurse. "No. I'm content, considering."

"Considering?" she responded, a scrunch of her nose and tightened cheek muscles creating a curious smile.

I pulled out of self-thoughts and looked up at the nurse. I decided to go for blunt. "A doctor told me I would need open-heart surgery. They explained to me that I had a heart attack and tried to describe that. Another doctor misdiagnosed me, telling me I had simply pulled a muscle in my back. I am content and thankful to be breathing, but my body has recently gone through physical hell." The words came out as though I was disciplining a five-year-old. "So, considering all that, I'm content."

"Jef!" Diana broke in with a directed, startled whisper. I immediately regretted my bluntness.

"But I am incredibly happy to have a wonderful nurse to help me recover. Thank you so much!" I knew I was back-peddling, and doing it badly, but I couldn't help myself.

My nurse's once-pretty face had tightened. "So, *you* are okay here." It was a statement, not a question, with the *you* pronounced with grit.

"Dandy," I responded, half-heartedly.

My nurse pretty much marched out. The door automatically closed behind her. There was silence in the room, and it felt perfect. I lowered the top of the bed slightly. Sleep found me quickly as I listened to an exasperated sigh and half-giggle from my wife.

It was my second day in the hospital. I was introduced to a potpourri of pills, IV injections, and grim looks of concern from friends and family who visited me. I was given thin manuals about the heart, cholesterol, fruits and vegetables, symptoms, blood pressure, and sex after a heart attack. I was instructed by dieticians, nurses, doctors, phlebotomists, and x-ray technicians as to what they were doing, how it would help, what I had to do, and what I shouldn't do. It was like cramming for a final in college while they injected me with more pharmaceuticals than any Haight-Ashbury hippies downed in the sixties. I was exhausted. My arms were tattooed with bluish-black veins from IV needles taped securely to sore skin.

After my diagnosis, I felt every beat of my heart and followed the current coursing through my veins. Every movement of my body was hyper-sensitive. If I peed, my bladder contracted, and the flow of urine was a force like a waterfall. I was fully aware, with deep sensitivity, of stomach acids attacking the food I ate. Any slight discomfort or natural process anywhere in my chest caused an explosion of paranoia. My senses were working overtime, and it was rather frightening.

I lay in my hospital bed, absorbed in my own physiology. I took each breath with a slight panic. Whenever I carefully rolled to change position, I anticipated pain that may or may not happen. I thought about life, and those reflections flowed unbidden into thoughts of dismal morgues. I had compassion that I hadn't had a week earlier. I was enjoying things as minute as perspiration and fingernails growing.

I thought about Kyle, young and ready to whip the world. What was he thinking? How had his tumor-infested mind dealt with a dad being locked away in a hospital and his mom alternating between hospital stays and treatment appointment? And what were my sons Jeremy, Jim, and Timothy thinking? My heart attack had a ripple effect that just kept growing. *A sick body is not a good thing to have.*

With a rat-tat-tat knock on my door, the surgeon, Dr. Thorn, walked in. He was accompanied by two "associates," as he called them—a Dr. Wilden and a physician's assistant, Dwain something. Dr. Wilden was a dark-eyed man in his mid-thirties. He kept his mouth tightly closed as he listened attentively; his long neck protruded from bleached green scrubs. His body slightly tilted on narrow ankles, and he wore no socks. Dwain had a gentle grin and a rounded chin. He looked like he was in his early thirties, but it didn't appear that he shaved yet. His striped shirt bulged with the shoulders and arms of a weightlifter or college wrestler.

My wife, with her attention to detail, had checked up on Dr. Thorn by searching databases throughout the country. She told me he was supposedly one of the ten best heart surgeons in the country considering long-term outcomes. That was a comforting thought.

Dr. Thorn carried himself well in what appeared to be a tailored suit. He had the erect stature and stance of arrogance. His words matched his posture. He was beyond surety; even his ego had an ego. Using two fingers to point at my chest and leg, Dr. Thorn explained bypass surgery. It was so matter of fact; I had the impression he was explaining how to overhaul the carburetor on my truck. It sounded as though the experience was going to happen to someone else. I was told he would remove several veins from a leg and attach them to the heart, which would increase the flow of blood to the heart. He concluded his lecture by saying, "You should be up and around within a day or two."

I did pick up several sobering facts from his diagram and pen pointing. One of my arteries was completely blocked. One was 70 percent blocked. One was 70 to 80 percent blocked. The fourth was partially blocked (he gave no percentage). He would need to bypass each of these, and perhaps a fifth. He said the surgery was extremely successful, with only a 1 to 2 percent death rate. Diana took notes on all the percentages. She loves this kind of talk. She would be making graphs and colored charts for my later enjoyment. Dr. Thorn indicated I would be in the hospital four to five days, and it would be six to eight weeks before I could return to work and normal life. Diana jotted down the timing figures, salivating for more numbers to add to the statistics she had found at the hospital library.

I didn't hear anything about the throat to sternum cut or the chest spreader. I wasn't told about the heart-lung machine. Dr. Thorn avoided explaining the loss of leg feeling and the pain of movement I would suffer afterwards. I already had enough fear and worry flowing through me to float any vessel.

It was oddly comforting that he was so sure of himself and so obviously full of himself. He seemed competent, as the nurses had told me. I was glad for that. I was prepared—at least on the outside.

As the idea of surgery settled into my mind, a calm descended on me. Life is reflective, and it was an awe-inspiring experience to be carried so close to death—not because I was afraid of death, but because I was amazed by the understanding and serenity that flowed over me. My first response was chest-tightening, mind-numbing fear. Then acceptance took hold, acceptance of both the surgery and the possibility of death. I felt I could deal with death—I didn't have much say in it anyway. It just happens.

They medicated me with drugs that slowed down my heartbeat and drugs that reduced the swelling around my heart. I was given lists of things to do and eat and do some more. They had decided that with all the sleep deprivation caused by the hospital, they were going to let me go home and rest up for my surgery there.

I was released the next morning. I was willing to wait while my body adjusted to varied pharmaceuticals and healing so I could have the heart bypass operation.

10

My own bed brought welcoming warmth when compared to the sterile disinfectant smell of the hospital. There was an unsaid sigh of relief in being home. Dogs barked in the distance, a motorcycle revved on the street, children screamed in joy, and all the familiar things lowered my pulse slightly. The internal fear about the heart attack still lingered in the background, though, like seeing an unpleasant acquaintance from afar and steeling oneself for its inevitable approach. An uncomfortable ember glowed and charred some unknown region in my stomach. It is interesting how we humans consider and reconsider things in our minds but feel the unpleasantness of our thoughts deep in our stomach. An organ that is physiologically so detached and far away is right in tune psychologically. I suppose God hardwired us that way, letting us feel caution, concern, and worry.

These fearful thoughts stay for years, only slowly retreating to the horizon of the mind until they are almost completely out of sight. Yet, they always remain as a faint, faraway memory. And even when fear is far distant, it can rush forward at any time. That is the real fear—the memory from real experiences.

I slept intermittently throughout that first day home, waking only for an input and output of water. The only rooms I saw were the bedroom and the bathroom, with lightheaded glances of a quiet hallway. I only felt my wife's presence; I cannot remember holding her hand, though I'm sure I did. I felt the comfort of her presence without my physical acknowledgment. I have no memory of her talking to me, although I'm sure she kept me company with her soothing voice. It would have been a good time for her to complain about me—to release her demons. After all, I wasn't exactly able to stand up for myself. But I know her thoughts were only loving ones.

I awoke at seven the next morning. It was Thanksgiving Day. *Ironic.* I didn't even care. Forty pilgrims in full black attire and the same number of Indians with buckskin shoes and full headdresses could have marched past me, and I wouldn't have even raised an eyebrow.

Diana fixed an adequate breakfast. I dug into it quickly but ate only a small amount. Through habit, my mind experienced hunger flares as I sat at the kitchen counter. My fork-to-mouth action, though, was more of an attempt than anything very productive. A ate few bites of toast, broke the yoke on the egg, and took a sip or two of juice poured lovingly from a paper carton. That was about it. Mostly, I stared at the breakfast and the kitchen with the vigor of a plastic houseplant.

I think I was a little depressed, though I really didn't realize it. I had never experienced depression, so I'm not exactly sure how it feels. I had seen it in textbooks and on television commercials but implying that I knew what it is would be like thinking you can swim because you saw a fish in a backyard pond.

The shuttle of nurses and technicians had ceased. A snowblower or two had replaced the beeping machines. There were no friendly dietary girls bringing me trays of almost recognizable food. Family and friends were not parading on their designated shifts. I had slept through the entire night without the interruption of blood letters, bicep cuff squeezers, and pill-dispensing shoulder shakers. There were no midnight wheels amplified on the tiles and big diagnostic machines.

You'd think that was a relief, but it was too peaceful. It was all too quiet. It gave me too much time to contemplate and prophesy about myself. I thought about the hospital and wondered who was on shift. Somewhere deep inside, I was missing cardiac care life. Where was the sleep deprivation? What about the twenty-four-hour construction zone? I was feeling a bit discarded and alone without all the prodding throughout the night. *Damn. When I come to my senses, this is going to feel pathetic.*

Thanksgiving was a big deal at our house. I love the smell of cooking the turkey and basting with skill and patience. I mash up enough potatoes for a regiment of marines. I flavor dry bread with chicken broth, celery, cashews, bird spices, butter, pieces of apple, and chopped onion; I knead it with my fingers until it is fully mixed and stuff it into the turkey. I cook beans and yams. Dinner preparation is a project I usually begin days before and savor days after.

At Thanksgiving, we have friends and family over. We have great conversations. We each recall tidbits of a memories and put each puzzle together with flying sentences. We all share stories of what has happened since the last time we met. Even the bad, poorly related stories are entertaining. We share what we are thankful for. Then we all disperse, satiated, after devouring disgusting quantities of food. And we are happy about the whole process.

I think Thanksgiving is my favorite holiday.

This year we had been asked to attend a couple of family Thanksgiving dinners. Diana and I had turned down the invitations, citing *cardiac arrest* as our reason. The *real* reason was that I felt like crap. The thought of leaving the house, going somewhere else, eating heaping portions, and finding the energy to converse was odious. In contrast, this calm, quiet, post-hospital time with Diana sounded so wonderful. I had no appetite for food or heavy conversation about all the facts of my cardiac arrest. I think Diana was also enjoying this one-on-one time together at home. Kyle was at his grandmothers feasting and the other kids were at their moms. Diana, like me was worn down from all of it.

For both of us, the time at home was a kind of recuperation from the reality of my stupid condition. We were both carrying a bag of rocks, knowing full well that in a few weeks I would re-enter the hospital for bypass surgery. That information was wedged way back in our minds, held tenuously by rotting rubber bands, and the anticipation absolutely sucked the air from our lungs. It was a thing to deal with later—not now.

The future was out of our control, and we could control only the immediate, so we basked there — joking and talking about lighter subjects, forgetting about rib spreaders and saline bags for a time. We skipped the weather (thank God) and discussed fond memories, people's idiosyncrasies, and our own funny faults. It was pleasant conversation.

My slowly reviving heart was good at that. It was weak enough to keep my boat trolling with no wake. I slept more than one should. I couldn't help it. Sleep was broken up by short, slow conversation and rest. I was a model for rest and relaxation. The handfuls of pills I took accentuated the fatigue, and my body followed.

I had off-and-on naps until about eleven-thirty, when the doorbell rang. I sat up, startled, lying on the couch. I stared at Diana. A sleep web of time and place confusion was woven throughout my head.

"Who's that?" I snapped. "Is it still Thanksgiving Day?" *Visitors. Don't let it be visitors. Why can't I have something scary and contagious that keeps people away? Damn cardiac crap.*

"I don't know." Diana whispered and blinked, trying to shake sleep from her eyes.

I slowly got up from the couch, clutching my chest over my heart. This had been a new reflex of mine since the word *heart attack* was mentioned. I grabbed my chest when I sat down. I grabbed my chest when I sat up. I grabbed my chest when I turned a corner. I held on to my heart when I coughed. It was an overly protective action, I knew, but I used it a lot. I headed down the stairs toward the door.

There at the door stood two, all-grins-and-giggles people from work. Both carried pots covered with tin foil; I could smell roasted turkey and vegetables. "Happy Thanksgiving," they both said as I stepped to the side.

I stood perplexed and dazed. I licked my lips to say something, but there appeared to be insufficient moisture to allow words to come out, even if I could have formulated them. *What the hell?* Shoes, wet from snow, padded up the stairs. Diana greeted them and pointed toward the kitchen. The smells were more powerful than the no-visitor policy I'd asked for.

I turned toward the open door. More friends from work wiped their feet on the door mat, entered with smiles and containers, and strolled up the stairs. The fragrance of homemade food followed, filling my house with its comforting, billowing aroma. A wave of euphoria lifted me while a winter chill blew through the open doorway.

"Close the door and come upstairs," said Diana.

Hosanna had floated that brown, basted turkey in front of me as she climbed the stairs of our split-level home. It was so big that the legs stuck out from the tin foil on each side. Other work friends wearing oven mitts passed me with a pan of potatoes and a bowl of gravy

I understood the gift of Thanksgiving that my colleagues brought, but I was immobilized by my awe. Friends brought food and smiles up the stairs and made kitchen noises as pans were displayed on the counter. My wife laughed between high-pitched expressions of thanks. I gained an immediate appetite as I half-way regained my composure and reached over to close the door. To my surprise, four fingers pushed the door back open.

Mike and his wife, Kim, stood in the doorway. Mike has a round, boyish face, on a large, soft body. We had worked at each other's side for a few years, acquiring a warm but tentative friendship. Mike held a bag of rolls; steam formed in the clear plastic bag as heat radiated from the bread. As I glanced past the two of them, three others were walking up the sidewalk. All had small burdens with familiar smells in outstretched hands. Mike and Kim walked past me with quick, standard greetings and lies ("You're looking good!") as they bounced up the stairs in cheerful succession. They smiled warmly, but I read their eyes: "Oooo! That's an odd shade of pale gray you're wearing today. Is blood actually circulating in that corpse?"

The other three were also friends from work—Janiel, John, and his wife, whose name I couldn't remember. Janiel was the secretary and friend who taught me all things biblical, answering my absurd questions with patience and warmth. No matter what she was doing, she beamed like a lighthouse. I could tell from the aroma that whatever she carried was chocolate—and sure enough, it was a German chocolate pie from Marie Callender's. Even though I'm not a chocolate fan, I loved the smell from the box that day.

John and his petite wife followed Janiel into my home. They brought a basket of fruit; a tinseled holiday bow was on the handle, and shredded cellophane grass cushioned apples, oranges, and bananas. John worked in delivery, setting up truck routes and calculating load sizes. He was wide, round, and cantankerous, but that day he wore a grin his face wasn't used to. His wife was a shy, tiny attachment—a pleasant, lithe lady, who faded in and out from behind him.

I had always thought of most of these people as acquaintances, but here they were, being friends—doing things for another person, not just shadows who greet each other at work. It was a social circle I was proud to belong to. I think very highly of the people I consider my friends. On that day, I added a few more to my list. By the time they were all in the house, eight visitors had passed me on the landing.

I took one more glance outside to verify that the parade had ended; I closed the door and climbed the stairs. There were hurried instructions to Diana about reheating, and a lot of people talked at once delivering get-better wishes. I was thankful no one told me about an aunt or cousin who went through the same thing. I had endured enough of that in the hospital. This day was filled with charming, fast conversation, perfect for the way my spent body was feeling and adjusting.

Like a gust of wind, they came and went. They left in the same order they arrived, almost as if they had planned if that way. During the departures, Diana took my place at the door. With a lump the size of a bulldozer in my throat and my heart thumping out of whack from the excitement, I stood at the top of the stairs waving politician-style at the retreating guests.

The lump in my chest made it difficult to breathe. I rolled over the arm of the couch and took slow, laborious breaths, trying to hold back tears. Diana sat down by me. We held each other, blubbering periodically. My heart held sturdy in the palm of my hand.

I went from crying to laughing. Diana looked at me with an expression of concern. "You okay?" she asked softly.

"They all said I looked great. They must be blind and stupid. I think the food smells got to them, too. I know I look as though

I've been on a three-day bender. I have a pain med hangover. My eyes are puffy. My cheeks are flushed. My skin is blue—I sweat from pores that didn't exist a few weeks ago. My hair is styled after Einstein. I move around meekly, with my palm attached to my chest. My beard is shaved like a corn maze. I think I've worn the same shirt for three days and three nights. My pants . . . look at my pants, they are those loose cotton workout pants that you bow tie to your hips. They look like I stole them from a thrift shop bin. And they said I look great. They are all going straight to hell for lying, pants on fire and all—definitely."

I started crying again. My eyes were glassy, my throat thick and dry. Diana patted my back. I shook her off. I needed to man up; but wow, it was hard.

She stood up, saying, "You're right, you do look like crap!"

I wiped my eyes and smiled. "Thank you. I feel like crap too!"

"Then you look how you feel, and you're dressed for the part." She paused and leaned over with hands on bent knees. What do you want to do now?"

"Let's eat all that Thanksgiving charity in the kitchen."

"Those are nice friends."

"Yeah, and those are the friends I don't even like." I smiled to myself, giggling.

Diana smirked, and we both went into the kitchen, laughing.

The Thanksgiving smells created a euphoria for hours. We ate and laughed at silly things. The two of us, alone, dressed like a third-generation welfare couple, had the best Thanksgiving I can ever remember. I have enjoyed a lot of memorable holiday turkeys, but this one tasted the best. It was made from friendship and thoughtfulness. I even broke my own tradition and said a blessing on the food. I have always delegated the prayer stuff to others who are more in touch with a heavenly being, including my wife. I wanted those kinds of people to make sure the food was okay. But I was feeling a bit closer to God. When He heard my short, pointed blessing on the food, I wondered if God scratched his head, saying, "I don't recognize that voice. Who is that?"

We were given a butter- and herb-basted turkey with mashed potatoes and thin, durable, peppered gravy. There was dressing; it was dry, made mostly of breadcrumbs seasoned with sage, paprika, and parsley, but it was flavorful. We were gifted with fresh green beans, a dish of yams baked with a punch of spice, and those fluffy, mushroom-shaped rolls. All the incredible, yummy foods were loaded with hidden, heart-stopping chemistry, and I didn't care. I had an operation scheduled to clean out my faulty plumbing. What was one more roll slathered with butter going to do?

The meal was terrific; each bite seemed more succulent than the one before. The two of us ate like Vikings. We hadn't realized how famished we were. Meat was ripped from the bones. Drinks were spilled. Spoons and forks were used simultaneously, going from plate to mouth with blurring speed. There was no need for napkins; we would spray off later. We laughed and giggled, blurting out half sentences only the two of us understood between bites with minimal chewing and harsh swallows. The dinner was fun. We were fun. I had forgotten to hold my chest; instead, I had a much-needed good time.

As with all Thanksgiving dinners, our meal ended with lethargy. We leaned back in our chairs, our stomachs filled with gratitude. Our pant ties loosened. Feeble noises were uttered with no need for response. A satisfied smile was the best we could do.

After what seemed like hours of satiated silence, I said without really meaning it, "Let me clean up."

Diana responded with a hollow giggle. "No, let me clean up."

Neither of us moved even slightly from our perches.

After another period of silence, I said, "Really, let me clean up; I need the exercise."

More time passed. "No, I'll clean up, and that's final." After several more minutes, she said, "Well, it was your friends from work. Maybe you should clean up."

The outline of a smirk formed on my face. "How about if we both clean up . . . you start."

Out of the corner of my eye, I could see her thinking.

"How about if we both go to bed and take a nap. Screw the dishes."

"Screw the dishes," I responded, and we both got up and headed for a nap.

My tiny mother and blonde, vivacious sister stopped by just before dark. We talked and laughed as I pillowed myself upright on the couch for visitors. They told me about Thanksgiving at my older sister's house. The food was abundant and the group smaller than usual. It was a formal dinner, with unlit candles and courses brought out in timed succession. They enjoyed the event, but all the food made them sleepy. It was pretty much the standard November gathering of food, exhaustion, and sleep, in that order. My mom, who had been losing height since she turned eighty, spoke about the wonderful view from the dinner table. Diana and I explained our gifted Thanksgiving dinner. We talked about how wonderful friends can be. Sometimes people know what you need even when you don't.

I received very nice phone calls from all my boys and a call from my elder sister, Annette. Diana and I visited with them all, passing the phone back and forth. I lay down and rested while she took her turn at the phone; then, when she gave me a poke in my ribs, I came to attention and conversed. We were quite a tag team. I slept deeply on the couch for two hours after all the visits and phone conversations. I never realized talking could be so physically draining.

Somehow, somebody cleaned up the dinner table and put things in the fridge. How long can turkey sit out? I wasn't sure, but I didn't want to take any chances. I asked Diana to heat up chicken noodle soup for dinner late that night.

My next few days at home were filled with Diana waiting on me, watching TV, reading books from friends stacked around the bed and couch, entertaining visitors with he-looks-like-crap eyes, rotating bouts of sleep and delirium, and picking at unfinished plates of food. It was a jail of sorts. I didn't have enough energy to do more than walk to the bathroom and bedroom or sit on a kitchen chair staring off into space like a sedative-laden, psychiatric patient. My mind was lax, so simple things like reading seemed to be a real chore. I was still shell-shocked from taking new medicines and undergoing the poking and prodding at the hospital.

I'm sure Diana was exhausted. She was taking care of my needs, working at her law office, running to pick up specialty pills for Kyle, taking Kyle to chemotherapy and various doctors' visits, fixing incredible meals, straightening the house after her slothful and lightheaded husband, and arguing with judges and clients. Her plate was full, and I was heaping more onto it. She was doing amazingly well under the stress.

A few sunrises passed, and I woke invigorated one morning. Toothpaste tasted great. My body was lifting out of its arthritic state, bending somewhat freely. I ate breakfast as though it mattered. I walked outside, where even the chill of winter felt good. I didn't stay outside long—maybe not even a full minute—but it was energizing.

Diana was asleep, but I had to wake her up to enjoy my sudden vitality. I shook her and received rumbling and a reflexive swat in return. I tickled her soft neck and shoulder, receiving a painful elbow to my thinly covered ribs. I was feeling too wonderful to let any of that deter me. I began blowing softly in her ear. The bed sheets found immediate life, hiding her in a twisted cocoon of covers. Waking her was going to be much harder than I'd anticipated.

I turned on the radio, full blast, and scurried from the room. I heard not-so-subtle expletives above the music, coming from somewhere below the sheets and blankets. I heard slapping sounds as Diana hit the table repeatedly, searching for the alarm radio. Once she hit the snooze button with a hard smack, there was dead silence. I wondered if the radio was still intact. I had been smart to leave the room with haste and wait it out.

I busied myself in the kitchen, preparing toast and strawberry jam. I poured a small glass of apple juice and another of tap water. With my newly found erect posture, I enjoyed my small but satisfying breakfast with zeal. Bread and sugared fruit had never tasted so good.

I was all better. The cardiac problems were healed. It was a new beginning.

The silence was pleasant, but I wanted morning conversation, an exchange of ideas and thoughts. I had a second wind powering my sails, and I wanted to untie and take off to unknown ports. I knew this feeling of well-being was just a short gust, and I wanted to take it somewhere—not idle it away at shore until the mainsail went slack, leaving me dormant again. I knew the wind would change any time now. My energy levels went up and down at the whim of some internal chemistry as my heart adjusted.

I took my medications with "tons of water," as I was told, then headed back to wake Diana, a slight snicker pasted naughtily across my face. I was feeling better—my sails billowed.

"Good morning, good morning, it's a wonderful day. The clouds are thinning. Get up." I was almost singing.

I paused, watching for a hint of motion beneath the blankets. The blinds were closed. There was nothing more than soft breathing and still hair. I leaned down closer to the top of the bundle that was wrapped tightly in bed sheets and blankets; surely, she was merely acting as though she hadn't heard me the first time. I tried a more demanding voice.

"Wake up! I am up. The world is up. You are going to miss a lot of wondrous things if you don't get out of bed this instant. The sun is up and shining—or at least it will be, when those massive, dark cumulonimbus clouds blow over."

"I'll manage. Now shut up and turn that light off." I recognized the strained lower voice of annoyance—she sounded somewhat satanic.

Next, I tried being sweet. "Honey, I need you to be up with me. I feel so much better. I'm cured. A miracle has happened. My heart has found its old rhythm. Listen, you can hear it beat."

" Go in the front room, and I'll be in there in a minute."

"I'm not four. I've played that with all the kids. I don't believe that 'I'll-be-there-in-a-minute' game. A minute becomes ten, ten becomes twenty, twenty becomes an hour, and so on. You think I'll just wait until I lose interest. Not happening, dear. Get up!"

"Really, just give me a few minutes to clear my head. I'll get up."

With complete distrust, I moved to the couch in the front room. I am not good at waiting. I hate lines at the grocery store, despise all attempts at receiving information from any government agency, and have no patience waiting for the mail or for my wife to do her hair. Sending me to another room created the same sense of anxiety.

After smothering my annoyance for more than the few minutes she had promised, I picked up a random book and began reading. It was a self-help book about coping with gardening problems. I don't garden. I never want to garden. I tried it and failed. Plants are better off with me admiring them at a distance, not participating in their growth and well-being. I am the angel of death to anything that contains chlorophyll. Plants turn brown just being around me. I do quite well with the plastic version, the ones stuck in moss-colored Styrofoam. My mom had the green thumb in our family. She could grow anything. She could nurse a limp plant to health like it was second nature. Her garden was vast, with colorful, stair-stepped flowers and perfectly trimmed bushes. She had a garden that produced tasty vegetables well into the winter months. The trees in her yard budded quickly, producing abundant apples, pears, and peaches; the blossoms perfumed the whole neighborhood.

It wasn't interesting for me to read about what my mother knew by instinct. It was a task, and my boredom grew with each word until my eyes slowly closed and my body slumped into the couch.

I awoke to the feeling of someone wiggling my earlobe. Diana's face blurred slowly into my vision.

"Want something to eat?"

Diana stood patiently by my side for what seemed to be five full minutes, though was probably only twenty seconds. My mind gradually re-entered our atmosphere. The hard gravity that was pulling me down slowly dissolved. I licked both lips and felt my tongue move back and forth across my teeth. They felt smooth and dry. I cranked my neck back and forth far enough to hear an inside popping sound. I licked my lips again.

"I fell asleep?" It was as much a statement as a question.

"I'm not sure you ever woke up. You feel like something to eat?"

"Tea and toast."

Closing my eyes again, I thought about my mother. When I was sick and in bed with annoying childhood illnesses like chicken pox and colds, Mom brought me toast and black tea sweetened with spoons full of sugar. It was her remedy for everything. If I had the flu, it was tea and toast. If a cold made my nose run and I coughed until my throat was sore, I received two slices of toast and a cup of hot, sweetened tea. When I had rheumatic fever as a grade schooler, tea and toast came to the rescue twice a day, sometimes more. Tea and toast covered pretty much everything except scraped elbows and knees. Then my mom, like all the others, resorted to a Band-Aid. As an adult, tea doesn't do much for me. But I do like toast, though now I want it dry, with strawberry jam and cream cheese.

"Tea and toast?" Diana questioned.

"Ohhh, no. Uh, how about a turkey sandwich and chips? . . . And, can it be on homemade bread?"

"Yeah, I'll get in there and bake up some bread first. Then I'll make the turkey sandwich. You're going to hold your breath for how long?"

"On second thought, I'll have whatever you're having."

"That I can do," Diana said with a half-smile.

11

I spent my days waiting for surgery reading, enjoying verbal sparring with my wife, and painfully trying to endure reruns and horrible news events on television. Diana and our kids cheered me up. Besides being a husband-and-wife team, we are best of friends. We can finish each other's sentences. Our intimacy is such that we laugh at jokes no one else would probably even get. Oh, we have differences—sometimes major ones—but those just seem to bind us with mutual respect. We also happen to enjoy each other's company.

Throughout the ordeal, our boys were always there for me. They didn't understand this version of me—a lethargic, couch-sleeping maggot. But like most maggots, I was eventually going to change into something and fly around the house. Hopefully not as an angel—if that was even a remote possibility for my afterlife.

Whenever my children dropped in on my new sedentary lifestyle, I gained energy and a full dose of happy. They were remarkable. They were also scared and curious. They tried so hard to be positive. They held within themselves the multitude of questions they couldn't ask, questions with answers they didn't want to know. I think my heart pumped just a little better whenever I felt their presence. I spent time talking to them and reassuring them about how much better things would be after the surgery. My voice and gestures sounded certain, but my mind floated in a sea of what-ifs.

Then there was that bright light of energy and smiles that Kyle continually beamed. Through all of his trials and medicines and chemo bombardment, he was always a positive force. He would shuffle off bouts of vomiting and headaches as if they were a circling fly in the air. His tumor hit a short-term remission, but it was still there behind joyful eyes, puffy cheeks, and a crooked grin. No matter how he felt on any given day, he wanted normality, he wanted to go to school each day. Kyle was the binding glue of optimism that gave our family affirmative reassurance.

Sometimes, relatives or friends came by. Those stopping over without being obligated were wonderful to share conversation with. Those who *were* obligated to come by asked how I was doing without concern for whether I even answered.

Two weeks was a long, long time to wait for a necessary operation. As the surgeon explained it during my hospital stay, there was urgency to the surgery, and I critically needed it. Knowing those two things, my anxiety shot through the roof. The days were stretched to mind-numbing nothingness. The TV blathered. I had cabin fever so bad; thoughts of ripping off my bathrobe and kicking a hole through the front room wall sounded better and better. I memorized the pleats in the curtains and every wallboard imperfection throughout the main floor. I mimicked minor sounds of the house, making creaking noises and drip sounds from my throat.

I was so bored that open-heart surgery sounded like relief. My eyes were bloodshot from reading. Torn pages and bent covers on stacks of books circled me with anxiety. I began to enjoy visitors and clung to their pant cuffs as they were leaving. I woke too early. I slept too much. I endured fear whenever my heart skipped an imaginary beat. I was starting to think I was laughing at things that didn't exist. I looked around and hoped there was not a hidden camera somewhere, filming my pathetic behavior. I needed the operation *now*. Please!

Diana used her time between Thanksgiving and the date of my surgery studying and researching. She investigated all the information she could find on heart surgery, heart attacks, life expectancy, physiological problems, holistic medicine, herbal remedies, and on and on. Our printer was probably gasping for air as she printed off internet information by the box load. I'm positive the heat from the printer warmed our home.

She recorded everything on yellow, legal notepads with arrows, circled words, sentences written in balloons, and unrecognizable diagrams. She analyzed statistics and organized data. It became her second occupation. But that's just Diana. She loves having a problem she can grab with both hands and unravel enough to give the person with the problem a never-ending supply of advice.

When her mother needed knee surgery, Diana had a thick stack of notes on orthopedic surgeons, their statistics, hospitals, and each hospital's statistics. She printed off graphs of every description. Diana rated the surgeons by years of practice, rate of recovery, number of similar knee surgeries performed, known surgical complications, and scrub nurse opinions. I teased her that she had forgotten to include shoe size and how clean the doctor's car was—though for all I know, she had those facts on a separate chart. Diana's mom followed her advice on the doctor, the hospital, and the rehab institution. Everything turned out well. Who knows how things might have gone without Diana?

In her process of overtime investigation, a lot of trees fell to allow me access to more intelligence on bypass surgery than I would care to endure in a lifetime. Bless her informational heart!

Soon, Diana loaded me up with information about herbs and shared charts of expectancy rates. I was informed I should take CoQ10 to improve my circulation, drop my blood pressure, better deliver oxygen and nutrients to my heart, which would make me feel better. She said I needed more garlic to decrease my cholesterol level by 10 percent and to keep the fats from depositing on the inner walls of my arteries. She said the antioxidant Ginkgo Biloba should be taken immediately to increase the blood flow in my arteries, capillaries, and veins and to reduce the risk of blood clotting. Oh, and I needed to take hawthorn—a pigment in its flowers, leaves, and berries seems to lower blood pressure, dilate blood vessels, and strengthen the heart. I interrupted, asking what color the pigment in hawthorn is. Diana abruptly told me that it doesn't matter a damn bit. What matters is whether it would work wonders on my heart.

Being a natural skeptic, I started to ask why the doctors hadn't prescribed all these remedies instead of the ones medical research had come up with. Instead, I stopped and held my tongue. It is not good to mess with Mother Nature or a wife.

I was given several names of holistic healers of supposed prominence around our valley. I glanced dutifully at a map with red- and blue-star locations. My head was spinning. Several times I feigned sleep. That didn't work.

I was relieved to learn that my surgeon was highly rated on recovery time and lack of after-surgery complications. Also, I was advised that my chosen hospital was ranked well for its treatment of heart patients. It all sounded like I was to have a pleasant journey in the operating room and through recovery. Disney-flipping-land, here I come.

But I still had another week to wait, during which I remained a reluctant, listening participant in Diana's didactic recitation of facts. Diana, of course, called it conversation.

I was lectured on cayenne, chamomile tea, and others. I became a mindless, head-affirming creature, like those bobbing dolls in the back windows of late-model cars. *Yes, ma'am, yes, ma'am* my inside voice said while my lips remained tightly sealed. I envisioned my stomach bloating on spices and teas and herbs then exploding in a green, leafy mess. It's the little things that get one through the day.

Diana went on about cardiac exercise and heart-healthy foods. The cholesterols were broken down into HDLs, LDLs, and triglycerides. She showed me schematics on pulse rate, vitamins, and even prayer. I was brought up to date on the newest holistic techniques. She was relentless. Most days, while she worked at her law office, I was left with various stacks of printed material, just in case I missed her earlier lecture.

At the end, buried in mounds of paper statistics, I was looking forward to bypass surgery. The true appreciation of her efforts would come later.

The night before surgery was like most since my heart attack. I couldn't sleep. I wasn't afraid of the surgery or death but of the unknown. I worried about my children and Diana and any effect this might have on Kyle and his never-ending therapies. I lay heavily on the pillow, turning in spasmodic, quirky movements every few minutes, searching for a restful position. Relaxation was as untouchable as the stars.

My mind raced at light speed through hundreds of people and events in my life, snippets of memory. I would stop and gaze at one every so often, and then, without settling, jump to another memory. In my mind, I saw people I hadn't thought of in years. Most of the names were gone—on the tip of my tongue, as they say—but the events were there and vivid, good times and bad.

I remember thinking about my mom's sayings and could hear her voice calling me. I was four houses away. She would use a Morse code vernacular. She would stand on our big cement back porch and give a short "Jef." Next came a drawn-out "Jeeee-ff-eeerrrrrr-yyyyy" in a wonderful sing-song voice. If I didn't respond, she kept it up until I came home. At that time in my life, I was embarrassed. After my Mom called me a couple of times, the neighbor kids mimicked her. "Jef . . . Jeeee-ff-eeerrrrrr-yyyyy" echoed in different children's voices, ringing throughout the neighborhood. My mom was famous for her call—and her homemade cookies.

The night before surgery, I went through a video in my mind of all her fun little sayings and inflections. They made my mom who she was. They defined her. One was, "Shit all Friday," and it would end with something like, "What have you kids done to this room?" I'm still not sure what that meant, but I knew it was trouble.

I watched another re-run of her sayings, "Quit acting like a Pap Akered!" This was not a term of endearment. She never defined what it meant, but in context we figured out it meant unkempt, crude, vulgar, and sloppy in dress and in manners. I was "Pap Akered" at least a couple of times a week.

The video in my mind rolled on to "You little shits!" It was Mom's favorite when we got caught doing something wrong. It was the universal term for bad. She would add a word to it if we were good. It became, "You *cute* little shits!"

I thought a lot about her during that restless pre-surgery night. My mom was a complex woman. She could clean the house at hyper speed and then sit calmly, reading voraciously from her stack of library books. She baked homemade bread, cookies, pies, or rolls every day. Some days she baked them all in addition to keeping the toilets sparkling, weeding the garden, vacuuming the rugs, making the beds, serving the dinner—and she still somehow made time to run races with me in the back yard. My cute little mom also had two heart surgeries and two brain tumor surgeries and bounced back as if it none of it ever happened.

I received my vitality and happiness from my mom. She gave me the inherited and learned ability to enjoy life and practically burst with positive energy—sometimes to a fault, but mostly in perfect rapport with the people around me. She taught me that we all have the ability to complain, but we Huntsmans choose to limit it. We understand problems, but not depression. Depression is a dip in the road for us, not a place to set up camp.

On the other side of the family, I learned friendliness and caring from my father. He taught me to not have prejudices, even though he grew up in a divided mining town, where Greeks, Italians, Chinese, Blacks, and Irish each lived in specific areas of the city. He introduced me to hard work and taught me the value of money. I worked for him at his automotive brake shop from age six through fourteen. I started out making fifty cents per hour and didn't get a raise for several years. It was Saturday work, and the broom I pushed was taller than I was. I also received a great Saturday lunch with my Dad at the coffee shop two doors down. Hamburgers and time didn't help buy my go-cart, but they did add character and memories and molded me into who I am today.

My dad was also a featherweight boxer in his early twenties, so I learned how to defend myself. He quit teaching me to box when I was twelve and I punched him in the chin a bit too hard. He held his jaw for an hour afterward, smiling at me the whole time.

Other visitors wandered through my memory that night—mostly figments and brief glances of aunts, uncles, youthful friends, and memorable neighbors, now long gone. Exhausted, I finally fell to sleep.

I woke up initially feeling pleasant. Diana was holding my hand, asleep next to me. The boys were at other people's houses who would take them to school. I woke Diana at 5:30. My pleasant feelings soon dissipated. Today was the day of my first surgery, and it was like waking up into a nightmare. The reality of the day kicked my heart rate up a few notches. The inevitable unknown is more frightening than the familiar events of life. I don't think a full night's sleep would have helped. Fear and anxiety enveloped me.

Today was my date with the pompous, data-spewing surgeon who, quite literally, was going to cut my chest open. I didn't like the guy, but I definitely wanted him to perform my surgery. He may have been totally arrogant, but he was also highly competent. According to my what my wife had learned through her exhaustive research, my surgeon had lousy bedside manners (as reported by his patients, who commented online) but incredible recovery statistics. I would take good stats over good bedside manners any day. He was chosen by the hospital and approved by my cardiologist to slice me, move veins from one place to another, and sew me back up good as new. *What the hell, I'll do it. I guess.* After all, I had gone without food or water after midnight for a reason.

I also knew that sometime after surgery, I would be forced to put on those double nostril prongs, with their behind-the-ear hangers. I will never get used to the plastic oxygen fangs. They tried to keep them on me in the ER. They are uncomfortable, they are annoying, and they tickle; they dry out my nostrils, and they wrap around my ears. I feel tethered to the bed with them because they get wrapped in the sheets when I readjust my head on the pillow. I have never liked anything shoved up my nose.

When I was in the emergency room, I pulled the oxygen fangs down below my blonde mustache. Then a nurse walked by and pushed them back in, telling me to keep them in before she walked away. As soon as she was out of sight, I pulled them back out. It was my only protest. My only revolt. Unfortunately, there was a steady stream of nurses and nurse's aides to jam the oxygen tubes in my nostrils and scold me. They didn't wear down. I did. My revolt was over. I endured hours of the things giving me discomfort and anxiety. Finally, I pulled them so they were half in, half out. It was hard to tell which they were, so the nurses left my nostrils alone.

Here I was, facing a surgery in which they are cutting open my chest—and I'm stressing about a nostril cannula in my nose.

I decided if I made it through surgery, a few days of nostril torture wouldn't be all that bad, unless they made me take an oxygen tank and a pair of those nostril routers home. Perish the thought. I felt sorry for the patients who needed that, and I hoped I didn't end up being one of them.

12

The morning was in the high forties, an uncomfortable temperature, with bright blue skies and drifting waves of leftover snow. Icicles hung like lace doilies from the roof. There was enough breeze to lower the temperature another fifteen degrees and redden my cheeks as I walked to the car. With my carry-on luggage filled with books, a change of comfortable clothes, a new set of blue-checkered pajamas (my first since I was five, although that pair was brown with guns and cowboy hats), and hunger pains growling like bulldogs in my stomach, I sat quietly in the passenger seat. My mind was scattered, not landing on any thought long enough to form more than a subtle, brief glimpse. I was neither worried nor settled. I had abandoned all my normal, lithe, animated self. I was like a wad of gum, stuck to a shoe, moving in the direction and at the will of someone else.

The gum and Diana shared a comfortable silence as she started the car and turned backward to pull out of our driveway, her neck tight and twisted. We could have been going on a trip to warm Puerto Vallarta, Mexico. We weren't. We could have been buckling up to head to the airport, destined for Jamaica. That wasn't it either. Our itinerary was Saint Mark's Hospital, the new vacation spot for this season. Such is life!

Black clouds circled the hospital like a warning. My hands gripped my knees, and I forced myself to breathe while gray exhaust puffed from the vehicles in front of us. Our turn at the patient let-out area finally came.

"Maybe we should circle again," I said.

"Just get out," replied Diana. "I'll park the car and meet you in the lobby."

"They look closed," I said without moving.

Diana raised her brow. "It's a hospital."

"I see people going in, but I don't see any coming out. Don't you find that strange?"

"It's six in the morning." Diana nudged me with her shoulder. "Out!"

The corridors were plain and unadorned on the way to the prep room. That's the room where they strip away all your dignity while shaving parts of your body only a porn star could want hairless. Then they dress you in an open-backed gown of nonexistent modesty. This costume has two sets of thin strings—one around the neck, and another pair to pull the gown closed at the waist. A towel would've been better.

Being first on the surgeon's table at six in the morning has its benefits. I didn't have time to consider a cancellation. The surgeon and staff wouldn't be fatigued by previous surgeries. The room's bacteria would be fully disinfected from the night before. My anxiety wouldn't have time to percolate. Despite all those positives, a herd of buffalo stampeded through my gut and a chill spiraled up my spine. Diana gripped my hand as if it was the last time. Our eyes gazed into each other. *What the hell was I doing here? Should we run back home to make sure the door was locked?*

I hadn't been in the bed even long enough to get warm when the gurney arrived. My bed was raised, and I slid over onto the frigid gurney. They asked if I wanted an extra blanket. I looked down at the thin sheet they had put over me, and I nodded. My throat was desert dry.

Diana followed my wheeled procession down one hall, up an oversized elevator, and toward the double doors. She kissed me goodbye. She was dismissed. I was not. I was pushed down another hall, through more doors, around a corner, and placed unceremoniously next to the wall by myself. "They will be with you shortly," the orderly said as he walked down the hall and disappeared through a door.

Within a few minutes, a tall man in scrubs patted my shoulder. He had a wide chin and a thin torso. His glasses rested at the end of a broad nose as he looked at my chart. He introduced himself with such a familiar name, but I don't remember what it was. Maybe he was a Smith or a Brown or a

Jones. He explained that he was the anesthesiologist and would be "putting me to sleep." I had already received something to relax me in the prep room. He probably could have told me anything, and I would have agreed. I was asked to count backward from one hundred as my IV was injected with something that whispered, "Good night." I don't think I got past "Ninety-ninnnnneeee . . ."—and that was the end of the bottles of beer on the wall.

Without my knowing it, I was soon under bright lights, splotched with antiseptic paint. By signed release, I was willingly having my chest cut open (hopefully with a new scalpel), my ribs sawed open at a place where they were meant to stay together, and instruments and latex hands probe the formerly virgin landscape of my weakened heart. *Invasive* and *vulnerable* would not even begin to describe it.

As I mentioned before, I worked as a surgical tech and an orderly during my college years, so I knew something about what was going to happen. I was familiar with life in a surgical theater.

My pompous surgeon would share light conversation with one of the nurses or his surgical interns. If the surgeon liked music, it would play from a boom box in a corner. The music would, more than likely, be conservative and soothing—no AC/DC playing "Highway to Hell." It would be one of the ancient classics, like Bach or Beethoven. The staff would anticipate my surgeon's every move. If they failed to, they would be quickly chided.

Dr. Thorn would be fastidious—not out of concern for me, but to boost his stats. I was completely fine with that. Either way, I would be operated on by a highly competent surgeon. I might not want him over to my house for dinner and conversation, but he was free to cut my chest any way he pleased. If you wanted a surgeon who was methodological, precise, and knowledgeable, Dr. Thorn was your guy. I knew he would do an impeccable job on my heart. If you wanted a surgeon who would hold your hand with deep empathy, I wish you luck.

Heart surgery was happening to me, and I was oblivious.

In the operating room, there is no such thing as a patient's modesty or self-consciousness. You are calmed, sedated, and plunged into a state of anesthesia created by the mathematical precision of pharmaceuticals and oxygen. The surgical staff could be dancing and singing with Madonna to "Like a Virgin," and you wouldn't know it. They could be doing all sorts of absurd things. I prefer to believe that they were solemnly, energetically, and knowingly working on repairing my heart. Making a better pump to move all that blood around. I knew things happened in surgical suites—jokes told, highlights of dates explained, fishing trips boasted about, and so on. But I was grateful that I wouldn't hear or see any of it.

During one surgery, years ago, I observed as an orderly, the staff bet one of the scrub techs that he wouldn't eat a glob of fat that had been removed from a substantial lady. The fatty ball was the size of a marble. The amount of the bet kept increasing. The scrub tech tossed the fat into an autoclave (which heats and kills any germs or diseases from instruments), pulled it out, and popped it into his mouth. He received about sixty bucks for that. Hardly worth it, but things happen in the OR.

As the anesthesia wore off, I heard far-away voices in a dream-like state. Neurons began to fire. An unknown voice prattled. Through the gibberish, I understood words like *tube* and *relax* and *pull*. Dry plastic scratched the inside of my throat. Right after "three" was announced, I gagged as an endotracheal tube was pulled from my throat. What happened to one and two? Tears of surprise and pain filled my eyes.

I coughed and raised my chin up to inhale precious air. I coughed more as someone held my chest and told me to breathe slowly. I regained my normal breathing through a sandpapered throat. Each dry, purposeful intake of air was measured in my mind and timed perfectly. I had a fear of not doing it right. After several minutes, the autonomic process took over. The sweat on my brow gradually evaporated, and I relaxed—eyes still closed, mind hazy.

Like nudging up a heavy garage door, my eyes opened. Blurs of gray and black swam before me. Diana and a nurse with blue scrubs and a tan face gazed sympathetically down at me. In the background, the rhythm of the machines serenaded me. Hearing evidence of my heartbeat as I felt the soft movement of my chest after bypass surgery was a comforting sound. The room was dark and restful, except for the beeping blue and green screens from the hospital computer and heart monitor. The tint of blue on the faces studying me was surreal. I looked for telling signs from the expressions before me, but I was too dazed and confused. I assumed I was alive.

I panicked as my parched throat began burning. I mouthed the word *water* several times. My vocal cords didn't appear to work. I tried again and again as Diana and the nurse leaned down closer and closer. Maybe I just *thought* I was speaking. My mouth felt like it was moving. Perhaps not. Finally, I managed a weak, "Water." I was so thrilled; I tried it again. A loud, but husky, "Water!" filled the room. The voice scared me. It startled the nurse and Diana.

The nurse leaned slightly forward and said, "You still have a lot of anesthesia in you. I shouldn't give you water yet, or it could make you sick." She smiled and walked away.

I whispered to Diana, "Get . . . me . . . water! I am dying of thirst."

Diana leaned down, "But, she said . . ."

"No, no, no. Get me water, now!" Each word burned my throat like hot wind. The panic increased.

I had never been so thirsty in my life. I had undergone several hours of open-heart surgery and the only thing that hurt was my throat. My imagination was on overdrive. I envisioned droughts; hundred-degree deserts, with decaying bull skulls in the hot sand; and water conspiracies conceived by mean nurses who smiled then moved on.

Diana left. After what I assumed was an extended conversation with the nurse, she came back with a paper cup. My mouth would have watered if it hadn't been so parched. "She said I could give you ice chips."

"Ice chips?" I forced out, with distaste on my face. *That's it. I bet her mother is very proud of her.*

Diana talked softly, "Okay, okay. Ice is wet. Just try it. But go easy."

Like a mother bird dropping a worm into the mouth of her hatchling, Diana dropped a sliver of ice into my open mouth. The ice chips tasted heavenly. They were incredibly wet. I put my hands over hers, grasping the cup, and shook more into my mouth. As they melted, I felt every drop slide down my scorched throat. I shook the cup like dice and received a tease of liquid. It was wonderful. She let me hold the cup myself. *What a big boy.* With a weak grasp, I held the plastic cup like a teddy bear. I felt accomplished. Handing the cup back to my wife, I laid my head back, beaming. I had won. The nurse had lost. I received water. My throat smiled.

The nurse came back to check on me. She looked at the machines and punched a few buttons. She added a few notes to my chart.

All at once, bile shot up my throat and onto my nurse's cleavage. After a couple of dry heaves, I threw up melted ice chips into a bowl that appeared quickly in the nurse's hand. Her other hand dabbed a towel at her blue OR top. Short upstarts, then nothing. It was over. It felt as though I may have coughed my heart up. I panicked. With an irritable look on her face, the nurse scolded me about the water while Diana wiped drool off my post-surgical face. The nurse told me she was checking my chest sutures and tubes. She let out a long sigh.

The drink was worth it. I was still beyond parched. I saw my cup of ice tossed into a stainless-steel garbage bucket. In my mind, I scowled, but my face didn't change expression. The nurse and Diana gave pathetic stares in my direction. Then their faces filled with the I-warned-you expressions.

Oh, wait? She said she checked my sutures and tubes. What tubes? I looked down. The nurse was pulling my blanket to the side. The nurse looked at me as though she knew a question was on my lips.

"I have plastic tubes coming out of my body?" I said in shock.

The nurse responded in a matter-of-fact way. "Yes. Yes, you do. They are for draining any excess blood around your heart."

"EXCESS BLOOD?" I said, my voice starting to raise, shooting pains scorching my throat.

My wife's concerned eyes went back and forth from me to the nurse. She didn't blink.

The nurse pulled the blanket back over me. She stated calmly, "It is all precautionary and standard. No need to get excited or worry at all. After surgery, blood may pool or seep. This way, we can drain it. The tubes will be removed later tonight or tomorrow."

"These look like the tubes I used to sell for garden fountains at my plastics company. They attached to small pumps. I know I'm pretty hazy here, but this can't be normal."

"I assure you, it is completely normal following heart surgery. The tubes are sterile." She giggled under her breath. "They are not garden pond tubes."

"Is there anything else they put in me that I should know about? How much are they charging for these . . . *tubes?*"

She grabbed her chin between her index and thumb. "The bypass surgery went well. We are going to get you up and moving shortly. You will be in a regular room within a few hours." Apparently done with the update, she asked, "How do you feel?"

She was good. She'd changed the subject, and I hadn't even noticed.

"I am nauseous, and I have a terrible headache. I deathly thirsty and my throat hurts. I seem to fade in and out of consciousness. Oh, and I have two sterile, Frankenstein-like, fountain tubes coming out of me that weren't there before."

She acted like she was listening. She released her chin, which she had been holding as though thinking about my every word. "You are going through the standard steps following surgery. But you seem to talk more than most of my patients. That's good, by the way. Jef, you will fall off and on into a deep sleep. That is completely normal. Also, an FYI for you, you have three tubes, not two. They are all for your benefit. Relax; in a little while, we'll see if you can walk."

I took a breath and fell asleep. I had no idea I was in recovery. I'm not sure where I thought I was. Post anesthesia is a series of knowing some things and not knowing anything.

Groggy, disoriented, parched, lissome, inanimate, sutured, and frightened, I tried to swim toward the voice. It was distant and hollow. I began to sense the pressure of a hand on my shoulder; it was light at first, then the grip seemed to strengthen. I moved slightly. I was strapped down. As I tried to move, skin and hair pulled on my forearm. Claustrophobia swelled around me. I forced my eyes slightly open. With a head full of mush and weariness, I gazed down at my binds of cloth and IV tubes. I had twisted my own spider web. A lady in blue scrubs with a blue-and-chrome stethoscope necklace helped untangle me as panic had me gasping frantically for air and freedom.

My nurse had a pleasant voice. "Careful, careful, let's raise this up. It's okay. You're all tangled in wires and tubes. There's that one; now let me get the other." She gradually freed my arms from bondage. First one wrist, then the other.

Relief washed over my body in a physical drain from head to toe. My breathing normalized. The nurse straightened the oxygen prongs in my nose. She brushed back the shower curtain of hair that perspiration had plastered to my eyebrows.

"You're back," she stated. "You have been in a deep sleep for an hour or so. We need to see if you can walk, now that your tubes are untangled. Do you know where you are?"

The gears in my mind ground slowly. I wanted to answer the question. I knew the answer but getting it to my mouth took a lot of lip licking and concentration.

"In the hospital . . . in the dark . . . I had heart surgery. Am I in recovery?"

"Yes."

"Can I have a glass of water?"

She smiled. "In a while. We need to get you up walking."

I looked down at all the tubes, wires, and connection tabs. I held my hands up and opened my palms. My mind was far from alert. I tried to think about walking, took a deep breath, turned my head, and tried hard to intelligently use my facial expressions to convey to the nurse what I was thinking: *You're crazy*. Her face was stern. She crossed her arms. I wasn't so sure about her change in attitude. She was going to make sure I walked. *Damn woman*.

I finally spoke again, taking slow breaths between each word. "Where is my wife?"

"She'll be back shortly," the nurse's mouth said, though her eyes and rigid stance answered, *Don't know. Don't care.*

Diana came back into the room as the bed was tilting upward. I tried a smile. It was like the smile you do after having a root canal. She stood just off to the side, eyes wide, lips thinned. The gurney lifted like it was raising a box with a doll in it.

My nurse had asked another nurse to help her. My bed made whirling noises as my feet were lowered to the floor. My shoulders slumped with the weight. I noticed a metal plate at the bottom of the bed, where my feet rested in parallel. The ride was over at ninety degrees. With nurses holding my shoulders and arms to keep me from falling, I stood erect like an unbalanced bowling pin. Diana watched intently as the bottoms of my feet began to take the weight of my body.

I heard my nurse say, "Okay, now just try to take a few steps forward."

I lifted my right foot—clad in one of those cute, blue, hospital socks—and took a step forward. My foot swayed in the air then softly found the floor. My left foot went into motion next. I was walking, if one could call it that. All the nurses shouted their congratulations. It was like a baby's first step. I thought they were going to get a camera, they beamed with such excitement.

I took three leery steps forward and three uncertain steps back. I turned slightly to look. I stopped, mounted once again on the metal plate, and with a push of a button from my nurse's foot, I was laid back horizontal. I got pats on the shoulder for a job well done. *Good boy*. They acted as if a fair number of surgical heart patients couldn't do three steps after surgery. I knew it had only been a couple of hours since my surgery, but I had certainly expected to walk if I lived through surgery. I had never occurred to me that I couldn't. That was probably a good thing. I had enough on my plate that morning.

After the famous three-step stroll, I spent time talking to Diana. Her voice was pleasant and reassuring. There is comfort in a known voice and its anticipated comments. I assume the drugs had me babbling incoherently, though she smiled at my every word. She told me about people in the outside world who were reading magazines and watching mindless, daytime TV in the waiting room. They apparently all wished me well. Which was nice, considering they were friends and family. Diana was discussing the highlights of the cafeteria. I was mostly at the nodding stage at this point. We talked about Kyle and how hard chemotherapy had hit him the other day. My pains seemed insignificant after that. After about ten minutes, the nurses dismissed Diana into the general population.

My memory recalls only tiny fragments from the intensive care recovery room. I assume I slept through most of it. Diana probably visited me numerous times, but with being bottle fed and drugged unconscious, I can't remember. There must have been purposeful signs I was getting better, because I was eventually taken off the bed lift and moved to a standard bed on the cardiac care floor. I later found out my new bed wouldn't lift me to a standing position.

13

Before my heart surgery, I'd rarely taken an aspirin or a Tylenol—let alone *two*. I considered two an overdose. I would have made a horrible drug addict. Yet now a nurse was bringing me a paper cup full of multicolored pills to take. My eyes widened. I was having trouble catching my breath.

One white, oblong pill on top stared back at me. It was as big as those African beetles I had seen in *National Geographic* and seemed just about as appetizing. One size does *not* fit all. My throat tightened at the sight. I thought maybe the smaller pink, oblong pill was doable. The red round one was no problem whatsoever. A blue one caught my attention. It had oddly beveled edges and was a deep blue, like a robin's egg. I shook my head. That shape wasn't about to slide down any throat of mine. The others were regular shapes and sizes, but there were so many of them! They all looked insoluble. A lump of fear hung in my chest.

The nurse stood impatiently with a cup of water held toward me in her outstretched hand. The meat of her pale arm dripped from her bones in weighted mass. Indifference filled her rounded posture. She wasn't heavy. Her muscles simply lacked adequate tone and tension from inadequate and sparing use. She had the look of wear and sleepless nights. She had a pleasant mouth, upturned just enough to make me think she was giving me something special. She wasn't.

I ignored the water. I tried to feign stupidity with a puzzled look at the very full cup.

With unhurried movement, she pushed the button to elevate my upper body. I tried to will her away. That didn't work. The cup of water remained right before my eyes. I thought, *No, thank you*. She was undeterred. She took my hand and wrapped it around the cup as if I was incompetent. My fingers went flaccid and my hand dropped to my belly.

The nurse glanced at Diana for help. Diana gave me her stern stare—like I hadn't seen that before. "Here, just pop these in your mouth and swallow them down with some water," the nurse demanded. She pressed the cup towards my lips.

I turned my head away. Without looking at her, I blew out air. After a few moments of silence, I swiveled on my side and faced her. In a determined voice, I said, "There are too many. I will have to take them one at a time." I pointed to the white beetle pill, crinkled my nose, and tightened the muscles in my face. "Except that one."

Her chin lifted and her mouth tightened. "It's easier if you do it all at once, but however you want to do it."

"Does the big one come in five smaller ones, so a normal throat can swallow it?" I asked.

She surprised me with a hearty laugh. "No. . . . It will go down just as easily as the others."

"And, it's made for humans?" I paused, showing a bit of my tongue between my teeth and tilting my head just slightly. "My mom used to have a saying about things that could choke a horse. This looks like one of them."

"Yeah, we only give it to humans and horses. It isn't as big as it looks," she retorted with a slight smile.

I was starting to like this nurse. "It's an optical illusion, then? Can you cut it in half?"

She pushed the pills and the water at me. "No, we cannot cut it in half. It has a coating and has to be taken whole. You realize you are stalling?"

"Quit being a baby and take the pills," said Diana. "Kyle takes more than that in one pop, and he's only fourteen."

"He's too young to know the dangers."

I could tell my nurse was getting tired of our pill conversation. Her soft arms were crossed. She straightened her posture, leaning back on one leg.

Frustrated, I pulled my tray closer, took the way-too-full cup of pills from her hand, and set it on the silver tray. After looking at the cup for several silent seconds, I poured the pills out in a line along the tray. I started at one end of the line. With two fingers, I picked up the one closest to me. I set the pill on my tongue and took a hearty drink of the water. The pill went down with the water. I did this with all of them, one at a time. The nurse refilled my water twice from the plastic pitcher. Diana giggled, and I shot her a look. The last one was the big one. The longer I stared at it, the more ominous it became.

I pushed it along the tray with my finger. I took a short drink, thinking about gagging on that gigantic, final pill. The nurse held her crossed arms tight by the elbows. She wasn't leaving until she had visual proof that I had taken all of them. Her eyes darted back and forth from me to the paper cup like a warning. I delicately pinched the pill between thumb and forefinger. I guided it to my mouth, placing it with precision at the back, so that nothing would be in the way. I didn't want it lodged sideways as it began its journey. It was pointed narrow side down. With a giant swallow of water, the pill slid down.

I told the nurse I had felt it scrapping my insides as it grabbed on the way down. She laughed and strolled out of my room. I was alone with the white beetle waiting in my belly. I wondered if it would ever dissolve. How long would those caustic stomach juices take to eat away at that lump? What was its half-life . . . ten years?

Diana clapped. "What a big boy."

I turned, ignored her, and feigned sleep. It wasn't too much of an act; I was tired most of the time during recovery.

Diana chuckled. "Okay, so you're going to let me win this one?"

She knows me so well. With our type A personalities, it's hard to let anything slide. Each of us wants to be the leader, the boss, the winner, the controller, the captain, and the chief. It builds an interesting dynamic in our loving, giving, winning relationship.

There are times I allow her to be the leader. Sometimes she does the same for me, but it pains us both to do so. It is a tooth-pulling experience, though a necessary one. We bend and adjust, or things would fall apart. We each have firm knowledge of each other's need to steer the plane. So, though we fight over things with words, it is a friendly exchange. When it touches outside the borders of affability, one of us backs down. At least most times. We find humor in our sparring. It grounds us.

I began to make snoring sounds.

"I know you're not asleep." She stood up and came to the side of my bed. She held my hand, all discolored from IVs. "There is one good thing about your surgery. You seem to let me win more. Hopefully, that will be a lasting change."

I increased the volume of my snoring. After a full minute of vigorous sleep noises, I turned toward her, opening my eyes in a squinting, light-adjusting way. I took her hand with my tube-injected, taped hand. It felt nice, but eventually, with slight movement, pain shot through my wrist as pinched plastic tubes and clear tape yanked at the blackened skin on the back of my wrist. I guess love does hurt. My eyes caught hers. I raised my eyebrows and blue eyes, trying to signal, *Whatever*. She responded with a smile, making me caress the moment with my recuperating heart. We held hands for a while before I dropped into a deep, happy sleep.

By the third day after the bypass surgery, I could stand, walk, and use utensils all by myself. I was ambulatory, as they say in hospital speak. The evening before, I had moved my IV stand around the rectangular track, passing rooms at an embarrassing pace. The wall paint moved faster than I did. I raced around with three other patients, all of us decked out in the same patterned gowns, sharing similar gasps for hallway air, as we made the one-lap mark and turned into our rooms. We nodded to each other, a hello—the congeniality of the zipper club, all of us members with matching chest scars of heart surgery from breast to button.

Previously, the first time I tried the full lap, I only made it to the nurse's station across the hall and back. It was amazing when I finally managed a slow stroll around the full hundred feet or so of industrial carpet of the cardiac care unit. It felt like such an accomplishment. The process of recuperation is pathetic at best. That first walk was a bit hard on my ego. It hurt to move one foot in front of the other like an unoiled robot. Each bend of adjoining bones rubbed, creaked, and flamed with pain. A couple of seventy-year-olds passed me by, pushing their IV stands as though it was no problem. I wanted to hide in my room.

Breakfast consisted of oatmeal, milk, a box of apple juice, and toast so dry it slid down like folded sandpaper—and it tasted like that, too. The TV droned on without sparking a glimmer of interest on my part.

Life was happening just outside my window. I could sense it. People were driving to work, listening to CD music and traffic noise. Children were sent off to school, carrying backpacks filled with kid sandwiches, math books, and doodled-on notebooks. Stores were unlocking doors and lifting their gates. Home furnaces were kicking on. Shelves were being restocked with cans of beans and bins of fresh vegetables in well-lit grocery stores.

As for me, I was sore and a bit lightheaded. I had a two-tine, hollow fork shoved up my nose to keep my oxygen level steady, and I was staring at dots that seemed to move around the ceiling.

I lay upright and still, listening to the humming silence of my room. With breakfast digested, pills swallowed, pulse checked by my morning nurse, Diana's hand holding mine with incessant mothering, uninterruptable murmuring from my bruised throat, insane pushing of the remote button for a decent channel that didn't exist, and muscle-tightening pain with every grinding bone movement, I looked toward the single window again, for an escape. Clouds eased by as slow as hospital time.

My bladder was full, but I held off until the pressure put the gauge in the red zone. I had to try to move this pair of legs that were strangely feckless and metallic—joints not rusted, but overtightened. Something didn't feel right. A few minutes ago, I was happily humming. Now everything was making me cranky. Where was the laughter and sarcastic joking I normally played in my head?

My joints ached, but my wired-together chest with healing tube holes felt fine. My leg muscles were tight and immobile. Oh, yeah, the surgeons ripped veins out of my legs and attached them to my heart, to make it *run* better. That explained my leg pain. But it still didn't account for the pain my arms and my shoulders. Maybe Tai Chi exercises would limber me up.

The pressure in my bladder was building. I scooted to the edge of the bed with a face crinkled in pain; drawn-out moaning burst from somewhere deep within. My appendages were unyielding. It hurt to straighten. It hurt to bend. I still had a full bladder and an increasing need to empty it. My teeth were clamped together so tight that I was afraid I was going to break them like chalk

Diana stared at me with a strained grin and Grand Canyon crevices above her worried eyes. She came to my rescue. Her hands helped bend and maneuver my legs carefully toward the edge of the bed. She pulled on my arms, lifting my back enough to sit up. Slowly, I inched my butt toward the edge of the mattress until I stood up, obliquely, with the bed as a buttress. She grabbed my elbows and carefully helped me to the bathroom. Joints wouldn't bend. I walked as though I had made a boo-boo in my pants. That wasn't the case. The cords in my arms rose in pain as I pushed the IV stand across the tile. Finally, through the door, I swiveled myself in front of the toilet, my teeth still miraculously intact. With painful precision, I urinated into the bowl while Diana stood on guard duty at the open door. I gave myself a slight smile as I watched normal-colored pee spin and leave my sight. I washed my hands, though it was hard to turn on the tap.

A weak "Okay" squeezed from my mouth. Diana came to my side to help. Grabbing my elbows again, she helped me return in the same awkward, webbed-feet way. I was out of breath as she leaned me against the bed, taking the IV stand from my grip. *What the hell is this all about?* My legs still moved like rusted metal. Pain was shooting through my appendages with each slight motion. With her help, I made it back onto the bed. After I paused and took some deep breaths, Diana lifted my legs onto the mattress. My face was flushed, my breathing quick, and a sucking sound escaped my jaws. I was exhausted not from pain, but from the physical exertion involved in simple movement.

My mind ran volatile and scared, trying to find relief from the aching reality. Inside, I was screaming, *What the hell?*

Outside, my face was locked in a grimace so intense I thought I might implode. Diana and I looked at each other without words. Her face was so intense that I wondered if her teeth would cut through her lip at any second. I was experiencing something so treacherous it escaped the scope of understanding. My teeth had been clenched until my jaw hurt.

I buzzed the nurse. The voice on the squawk line told me there was a change of shift and the nurse would be there shortly. At the time, I hadn't realized "shortly" meant "never."

After twenty minutes or so of complete stillness, the pain subsided to a tolerable ache. I became fearful of moving any limbs. I relaxed my upper torso and arms in a Hindu yoga way. I could move them slowly without causing pain. From the hips down, the twitches and spasms in my legs subsided the longer they remained immobile.

Within an hour of my robotic duck walk, the physical torment had finally ceased. My skin on my face and neck had relaxed in stages. I fell asleep soon after with Diana massaging the muscles of my legs. My sleep was short but very needed. I awoke mildly incoherent and numb-headed. Surgery does that, or so I was told by my nurse and several visitors. In the hospital, there appeared to be no end to the moving line of people who were masters of the obvious.

Two taps sounded on the door. Through slits of eyelashes and sand, I saw my surgeon walking into my room. As always, he entered as if he were leading a brigade of soldiers into battle, a man of purpose—shoulders back, spine straight, chin out. A blurred figure followed him. I shook the drowsiness from my head. Now, instead of half-asleep, I was dizzy and lightheaded.

Dr. Thorn wasted little time. His arms were animated and his face stern as he explained how well the surgery had gone. As he spoke, his hands seemed to be typing on a three-dimensional typewriter, his fingers moving in sync with each word. All sentences ran together as one. He told me that my heart functions were stabilizing and something bad in my blood work was dissipating. As his arrogant explanation of my good health unfolded, it was obvious he was quite proud of himself. Most of his sentences started with "I did" and "I performed." After a while, he stopped.

After a period of awkward silence, I wondered if he were waiting for a standing ovation and a toast to his skilled mind and hands. Before I could applaud, he began again. He told me the things I could do to help my body begin healing, to eventually improve my life. That was helpful. His second-in-command stood behind him and nodded in obedient agreement, his right fist balled up under his chin.

Dr. Thorn wanted me to get up and out of bed and walk for him. I was ready to take a walk, but I felt like a circus dog as he hurriedly elevated the head of my bed. I turned to sit on the edge of the mattress. I had momentarily forgotten about my earlier, painful waddle to the bathroom. I barely moved before my body was immediately consumed by pain and something that seemed to be to be rigor mortis. I knew I couldn't have both at the same time—pain is for the living, and rigor mortis is for the dead. But that's how I felt. It had come on suddenly. My joints would not bend without great effort and anguish. My elbows and knees and spine flexed again like rusty hinges. Sleep seemed to have relieved my early morning walk of pain. Now it came back accompanied by an evil brother.

I was struggling to get up. My teeth ground as shooting pain radiated from my joints. Small, slow movements took my breath away. I moaned as my feet hit the tile and my butt rested on the bed. I stopped to catch my breath and let my muscles relax.

Apparently, I wasn't getting up fast enough for Dr. Thorn. He looked irritated that the process was taking so long. The doctor pulled me toward him by one of my sore arms and an unbending elbow, forcing me upright and forward. The torture throbbed through my body as I moved, step by step, with him, arms outstretched, yanking me toward the door.

"You need to walk," he ordered. His voice gruff and brutal.

I replied emphatically through tight lips, "This hurts!"

"You are just stiff from too much bed rest. You need to be up and moving to get better," Dr. Thorn scolded. Without any courtesy, he yanked at my arms.

I followed his grip as he jolted me through the door. Stiff legged and in excruciating pain, I was led ten feet from my room.

"Now, keep walking; you will feel better," he told me. He stood, let go of his grip on my arm, crossed his arms, and watched me, as if I were a trained pony being whipped into shape. He called out orders as if he were the drill sergeant of ambulation, coarse and indifferent. I wasn't about to give him any veneration.

As I forced myself to walk for the son-of-a-bitch, Diana helped by holding my elbow. I had a fund of expletives for him that filled my head on a rotating basis. I moved with tremendous stiffness and pain. My jaw clamped and my lips sucked in against them. I felt nothing but contempt for my surgeon, though I kept the pace up for one full lap and part of another, until he was out of sight behind a wall. We then moved through a nurse's station to the other side of the hall where my room was.

Dr. Thorn was gone, probably insensitively punishing another patient. I listened for screams, but the only ones I heard were locked in my own mind. Back in my room with Diana's help, my feet slipped closer to the sanctuary of my bed. I never wanted to wander into the hall again.

An interesting thing happened later that afternoon that shed new light on my condition and contempt for my surgeon. It came to me and Diana as though God was sending a message through the electronic box mounted above our heads. The TV showed a commercial for Zocor, a cholesterol pill I was taking. There were images of people playing tennis and others walking on a beach, hand in hand. The scenes were softly lit and happy. After they emphasized all the wonderful benefits of Zocor, a quickly read script of the side effects announced, "In some individuals, this medication may cause pain and immobility in the joints. In the unlikely event this happens, immediately stop taking the prescription and notify your doctor."

Diana's eyes and mine were glued to that message. My pain and lack of movement made sense now. I wanted to punch the surgeon, if only I could make a fist.

We went through all the "he-should-have-known" comments. Then, just as my wife was going to have the nurse page my sadistic surgeon, my cardiologist, Dr. Vandoven, walked in.

"How are you feeling?" was his first question. It was wonderful to hear the concern in his voice and see a genuine smile fill his whole face.

One word came out of my mouth: "Zocor!"

He answered, puzzled. "Yes, Zocor. That's the statin you are on."

Diana explained to him about my aches and pains, my efforts at walking while Dr. Thorn impatiently pulled me along, the TV commercial, the side effects of Zocor, and how I needed to be off that medication right now. Dr. Vandoven agreed. He explained that I must be the one in a hundred people who experience these painful side effects. He empathized with my pain. He scribbled notes in my chart and talked to the nurse and said he would be back later to check on me. He assured me I would not receive Zocor again, and he would decide on another cholesterol-lowering drug after the effects wore off.

I felt much better. There would be an end to the agonizing paralysis. I was hoping the drug wore off quickly.

It is not good for the rehabilitation of a patient to find out the authorized prescription is basically poison to his system. It stagnates the confidence one hopes to have in the hospital. It cuts away at one's determination, like warm rain on an ice-cream cone. These things happen in life. I just wish they wouldn't have happened to me.

Always listen to your body. Sometimes it lets you know what's happening inside better than any doctor.

The foundation of Jef is built upon two basic principles: One is to take life lightly. The other is to laugh at myself. When a right hook loosens the jaw, when my lips are beginning to swell and darken, and when blood shoots through my battered gums and detached teeth, I chuckle at my inadequacy. Then I power an uppercut to my opponent's unpadded chin, adding a few solid jabs to the midsection until self surfaces, with nothing more than a sore face and an amusing story for later years. At the time, I found no joy in Zocor. Now, years later, I can find humor in its battering.

After Zocor, I was given Baycor, another statin drug for lowering cholesterol. As irony would have it, Baycor was taken off the market a month after I started using it because of its own list of adverse effects. As time went on, I tried a few other statins with minor debilitations to me until I was put on Crestor. Crestor worked for me without causing any reactions. Through this experience, I learned that each person is specific in some ways. The things that work for one person may not work for another. Finding the perfect mix of medications is a matter of trial and error.

Life has two intertwined, competing goals—obstacles and achievements. My philosophy is simple: don't wallow in the obstacles or boast of the achievements. All of us have both. They are two sides of the same coin. One does not come without the other. Grasp both firmly in your mind and spirit, using each to climb the stairs of a fun, enjoyable, full experience of life. We learn from each. We should laugh with each. Crying is an okay response, too; just don't take down the sails. Obstacles and humor about them ground us; they make us reconsider ourselves and our goals and create a base of bricks, not sand. I believe obstacles should build strength. Yes, this or that is hard on us, but learn from it and don't accept defeat. Just change course, and achievement will come in time. Then give it a little time and laugh about the problems.

A laugh or a grin is better medicine than any your doctor can prescribe. And it costs less, too.

Some of our greatest achievements evolve from blind luck. Others are formed by a hard, sweaty workout. Usually, it is a combination of the two. On the other hand, most obstacles are served to us by our own hands as our mind rests on the problems of a problem instead of on the solutions. There are also those uncontrollable, spontaneous obstacles and achievements that we must simply hop over or hop on, tip our horns down, and barrel through until the ride is over.

Nearly all experiences are humorous if you shine the light a certain way. Study each situation with squinted eyes. Taste it with childlike anticipation. Savor it with a mischievous giggle and give thanks for the experience. Smiles and laughter help. Life shouldn't be that serious. I know I'm not immune to bad times; life is incredibly serious and horrid at times, but perseverance and humor can at least improve one's attitude about the various facets of life.

I look at survival and existence this way. I have levity and buoyancy, whether the sun's rays are at my back or rain is drizzling down my neck. My attitude keeps me from visits to people with questions of a Freudian or Jungian nature. I believe verbally spilling out my inner self to a stranger is nuts, anyway (there is a reason we have true friends). I understand a good attitude doesn't work all the time, but it keeps me happy about 85 percent of the time. I fully believe a positive attitude creates health. Since my heart attack, I think it is one of the main things that has kept me out of a brass urn.

I realize that with my inner makeup and my attitude on life, I lose a full understanding of things like depression and self-pity. I have never had them. I'm not totally exempt; I visit bleakness for brief moments, laugh sadly at myself for indulging, taste the bitter flavor, and resume dancing down the yellow brick road. I just cannot find the time to be depressed or indulge in regretful, sorry feelings for long periods.

Something I do know about is the Cardiac Arrest Syndrome; it's when the sun brings out colors you never noticed before now that you have faced death head-on. My whole outlook changed. I find pleasure in things that were innocuous before. I have gained an eye for birds, bugs, leaves, and faces that I never had before. Anyone who has beat cancer or made it out of a car accident or escaped any situational death threat fully understands this syndrome. I certainly received a luminous truckload full of the sunny joys of life after recuperation. But then, I have always had a healing number of yellow-smiley-faced days woven into my DNA that were taught to me by my mother, who wasn't afraid to smile, laugh, and giggle. So, I take life's serious moments lightly and enjoy as much of the ride as possible.

Luckily, the Zocor effects had worn down from debilitating to just mildly inconvenient within a day. I took a deep breath of contentment, for once grateful that the government makes drug companies explain the risks of their remedies. I also thanked God that Diana and I happened to be watching television at exactly the right time.

There's a lot of trial and error in physicians' offices and in hospitals. Medicine is not an exact science. Remember, things that work for one person may do nothing for another—or, worse, the treatment could cause blistering hell. I have found this to be true time and time again.

I saw Dr. Thorn one time after the stiff-man-walk-of-torture incident. He never mentioned it. He never apologized for not recognizing a well-known prescription problem. He did mention how well his sutures were mending and what a positive future I had as a result of his surgical expertise.

I finally asked him if he had heard about my reaction to Zocor—how it froze my muscles and caused excruciating misery, and how it had kept me from walking for him in a normal way.

"Yes, I bet you're glad that was discovered," he said. "That was highly unusual."

I wanted to tell him, *Thanks for the death march. You would have been a hoot at Auschwitz.* But I kept my mouth shut, even though holding back caused my stomach to churn. As I learned firsthand, Dr. Thorn is an excellent cardiac surgeon but like all of us, he can make human mistakes.

Dr. Vandoven released me from the hospital the next morning.

"Released" may sound quick and easy, but it takes several hours—four hours and ten minutes, to be exact. There was a lot of waiting in between each step. A bundle of paperwork needed to be signed by me, the doctor, the attending nurse, and the lady who waters the plants. Prescriptions were handed to my wife, with both verbal and written instructions for each. I was given a cardiac packet that included pamphlets of every description on cardiac care, plus others with pictures and information on the surgery and the wonderful patient care that I received from the hospital.

The nurses and staff were incredibly helpful, as they put up with me. Tape was removed, along with a healthy dose of arm hair; IVs were quickly yanked from my veins. I glanced at my purple and bruised arms—the tattoos of a hospital visit. The sting slowly disappeared. It was amazing what bittersweet joy came from a simple thing like losing my bondage to tape, tubes, and collapsible bottles of liquids. Monitors were turned off and many old, sticky, square tabs were jerked from my chest, taking with them a slight layer of skin. I realized my profound gratitude that they had shaved my chest prior to surgery.

As my skin stung and tingled in various places, I bit hard on my bottom lip and gazed at my new scar. The long vertical chest scar is known as "the zipper" to most cardiac patients. It forms a camaraderie of friendship among all who bear it. It's like the friendship marines share. *Oorah!* Each group has its own set of battles and battle scars. All surgical heart patients have that strip of white tissue indicating ribs once spread open and making us feel unique. The skin feels different, and it creates a visual reminder of the fright-filled invasion. We weren't awake to see it happen, but we have deep perceptions of a violation done inside our bodies that was very necessary but not normal.

After all my belongings were packed in organized, plastic hospital sacks, Diana and I sat on the edge of the bed in silent anticipation of the wheelchair ride. In all hospitals, patients ride in a wheelchair from the Stryker bed to their awaiting car—it's the rule and a thwart to lawsuits. The obnoxious TV mumbled in the background. Other patients and staff padded down the halls, getting their exercise. We sat. We waited. We were told it was policy and for our protection. In truth, though, I'm certain the hospital doesn't want me passing out and gashing my head on the way to my car. After the designated thirty to forty minutes of biding our time, the wheelchair arrived with my assigned nurse's aide. There were smiles and relief all around. I was glad to leave. They needed the bed. And I needed to get out of it.

Leaving the hospital sounded incredible; going home sounded even better. The excitement of being homeward bound increased the pace of my heart. I was getting well just from the thought of it.

The obligatory chit-chat followed us down the hall, into the elevator, around the corner, and, with a swish, out the door. Diana pulled up in her car as the wheelchair and I hit the sidewalk. I was told I could walk to the car now. Good to know. I was not as steady as my mind thought I would be. I was dizzy and a bit nauseous; my weak, rubbery legs were not responding well to forward motion. Like a drunken Charlie Chaplin, I made it to the open door, dropping and spilling like a blob onto the seat.

As we drove away, relief settled over me. I had escaped. I was out. I had made it past heart surgery and all-night awakenings by nurses in Bugs Bunny scrubs. I was free!

14

Recuperation sounds like a positive, invigorating word. Say it slowly: Re . . . cup . . . er . . . ation. Listen. It sounds like a word describing the ancient hatching of an egg after which a perfect specimen that glows with inner essence crawls out.

Not even. Recuperation is extreme work for little gain. It's like being on an elevator with the door refusing to open. Stopping on floors as you go up and down, endlessly getting stuck on certain floors way too long. You keep pushing the door-open button on the higher floors, but the effort drops you back down toward the basement and then a basement below that and another below that. They—doctors, nurses, hospitals—don't let you know recovery is frustrating, with microbial wins and galactic losses. It's their dirty little secret.

A few weeks after chest-spreading surgery, weeks that seem like eternity, the elevator finally opens on a mid-level floor. You walk out, thrilled to have arrived somewhere. You become accustomed to the level you're on, hesitant to get back into the elevator to try the next floor up. Each one above the other means a longer stay. Sometimes, you barely make it inside the door, only to drop a floor or two. Such is the recuperation process. "Seventh floor, please. No, no, not the fifth. Oh, crap, why are all the lights blinking? Help!"

The house seemed quiet and unused. When I talked, I thought I heard a slight echo. Home was quiet and clean, with everything in its designated place. I figured it wouldn't take me long to ruffle it up a bit. It was a relief to wander aimlessly around the house at my slow, determined pace. It was peaceful and warm. I was only gone four days for the surgery, though it seemed an eternity. I lay down on the couch. Diana arranged pillows behind my back. This pampering was nice, too, even though I knew it would fade. I could almost hear *get it yourself* way off in the distance. But I determined to enjoy being cared for, while it lasted.

The front door slammed. And slammed again. Like loading cows through cattle chute, rumbling stormed up the stairs and turned the corner near the couch. Just when I thought my kids were ready to pounce on me with a welcome, they stopped short. Faces happy to see their dad but wondering if I'd break like a teacup. I sat up and motioned them to the couch. They bounced on both sides of me. The last time the boys had seen me I was wrapped in tubes, surrounded by beeping whirling machines, looking ghostlike, and trying to act as if everything is normal.

The reunion went well, but I was worn down quickly though I never let on. Once they realized I was going to be okay, they went back to being teens—food, Nintendo, and more food. They truly boosted my moral even though I didn't have the energy to show it most times.

Those first couple of days on my own couch were comforting. Lounging was about all I could do. Prescriptions made me content. Diana took care of me with loving grace. The boys spent the days at school. Kyle's cancer was staying even by drugs, radiation, and prayers.

My only exercise consisted of visits to the bathroom and the kitchen. Even with those short walks, my breathing was labored. Oh, and the expert shuffling and fluffing of pillows and readjustments to horizontal posture was an aerobic workout all its own.

My so-called relaxed comfort was short-lived. It didn't take long for boredom to set in. Boredom is an animal of headaches and irritability. I have never had any real fondness for sitting still. Inactivity has always been abnormal for me. My world imploded, and I grew fangs of nervous energy as the television slowly turned my eyes square. Books that were once sources of happy solitude became rectangles stacked up on guard duty, emphasizing my immobility. The couch was my prison. Breaking free was foremost on my mind.

Once I mastered the obligatory channel changing and couch pillow fluffing, I decided to try walking outside. I had to get away. Anywhere would do. The walls had turned to iron bars. I knew my way from the couch to the bed, and I had traveled into the kitchen a few times, though I seemed to be eating regularly on the couch. The crumbs of my existence were mounting. I realized I needed to breathe in the fresh, cool air of December. I needed real movement, not just shifting from pillow to pillow. When the walk to the bathroom and back is your only exercise, it's time to expand, before your routine narrows any more. I knew it meant lightheaded ventures, but I needed blood circulation. Dr. Thorn was right about one thing: I needed to walk more.

I was also losing any fashion style I may have once had. I half-jokingly acknowledged to Diana that my one pair of pajama bottoms and my two t-shirts—a Kenwood and a Puerto Vallarta toucan—should be taken out and burned. But there is something comforting in sameness. I bathed every day, changed my boxers, brushed my teeth, combed my hair, used musk deodorant, and put on pretty much the same outfit as the day before. Only the t-shirt, the TV channel, and my bookmark changed. I assumed Diana cleaned my two t-shirts, though I'm not sure I paid any attention.

I looked in my closet. I had fifty-plus shirts and at least fifteen pants hanging there. Yet, when I glanced across at the wall mirror, at the pathetic creature I had become, the same colorful toucan stared back at me with the words *Puerto Vallarta* printed beneath. The new morning stain above the bird was the only thing different. *No wonder I'm sick. This recuperation is not going well.*

This new beginning, this walking day, had begun like others. I brushed my teeth and combed my hair. I followed my ritual of pulling up the pant legs and centering the stretch band of my comfortable, once-new pajama bottoms. I sat on the couch in my Puerto Vallarta shirt, surfed television stations with little interest, and waited for Diana to arrive home from work. She had told me not to go wandering outside without her. Knowing my breathing capabilities at the time, I didn't argue. For once in my life, I wasn't all that sure of myself, anyway. I was all set for couch time with expletives on my breath, though I was determined to change my clothes before Diana got home. I wanted to take a real walk with her, hopefully one of several miles.

Periodically through the day, I did stretches and exercise. I moved aimlessly around the house in a determined, crouched-over stroll. I thought about doing sit-ups, but looking at my chest stitches, the fear of seeing my own lungs popping through parted ribs made me toss that idea out. I kicked a basketball around the room for a while. I stopped when the ball hit a table and ricocheted off the corner lamp. Our sons had rules—no soccer in the house—and here I was, thinking it was okay for me. "Do as I say, not as I do," I muttered aloud, a touch defensively. I also tried leg lifts, but that pulled at my chest stitches in a bad way. I stuck with aimlessly walking about the house and resting three times as long as I walked. Everything ached. With a moan, I slept for many, many hours until the phone woke me.

After my wife's call to say she was on her way, I got up and went to the bedroom. I found Levis I had worn in my pre-surgical era, folded nicely in a drawer; an ironed shirt; and tennis shoes with a thin coat of dust. I blew the dust back into the closet for safe keeping. I began to get dressed. I was finally stepping out of the elevator on a new floor. I started out in a hurry, as though late for an appointment, and I ended up panting between each finished shirt button. Slightly dizzy from an overworked heart, I took the shoes with me to the front room and collapsed horizontally onto the couch. I felt the remote pressing into my spine and didn't care. I relaxed for twenty minutes, which turned out to be almost an hour. My body slowly regained its remote-button-pushing stamina, though the remote lay beneath me untouched. I slipped on my tennis shoes with my feet in the air, tucking the laces into the sides. Tying shoelaces sounded frivolous and tiring.

I sat upright, breathing purposefully as I watched my buttoned shirt rise and fall with the motion of my lungs. Daytime was quiet and still. The silence was broken only by the refrigerator generator kicking on, then by the furnace pushing stale, warm air through the ducts. I stayed relaxed, feeling good about being dressed in real clothes. It was all reassuring. Recuperation.

I worried about Kyle through my slow recuperation. I couldn't do much but give him hugs and listen to his recap of his school day. Diana was taking him to radiation 2 to 3 times a week. She was being a super mom and a super wife and squeezing in a stacking workload at her office. I didn't realize all the balls she was juggling until months later. She's amazing.

Diana's on her way home usually meant she only had 320 more things to do before she left work. I was used to it. That doesn't mean I didn't get anxious about it at times. It just meant that twenty minutes means an hour to ninety minutes in Diana's reality. I adjusted for that; I always have.

I'm not sure how long I waited, nor did I care. I probably fell asleep for a time. I was a master at sudden unconsciousness. Diana eventually walked through the entrance and up the stairs to greet me. There was a kiss, a stare at my outfit, a smirk, and an unsure giggle.

"I want to go for a walk outside today," I announced.

"Really? Okay!" Diana smirked while she kept bobbing her head.

"No smart-ass remarks about my permanent couch exercise? Or my NEW recuperation line of clothing?"

"Hey, I didn't mean anything by that couch-sit-up remark I made last night." Diana's eyes smiled. "Let me change out of this skirt and heels, and we'll take a walk."

After she was in the bedroom searching for clothes, I called out, "You didn't say anything about what I'm wearing."

Diana walked back down the hall so I could hear her. "Trust me, I noticed. I've been waiting for a time when you might leave your hospital recuperation outfit here on the floor. These items will be in a garbage bag quickly, along with the gloves I plan to wear to pick them up."

"Ha! Don't even think about it. I'm already having separation anxiety. I'm thinking about opening a line of recuperation-wear outlets."

"That would be great. You wouldn't even have to iron them or put them on hangers for display," she said, enjoying herself. "Just dump them out of boxes onto tables. Oh, yeah, I forgot—Goodwill beat you to it, but theirs are less used."

"You must have been beaten up pretty hard at work today. I guess it's my turn now, huh?" I teased.

She deliberately ignored my humor. "Well, the clean Levis look great for a change, but I can see the same old t-shirt on under your blue shirt, and you're still wearing those worn-out moccasins, Pocahontas."

"First of all, Pocahontas was female. Second, these shoes are comfortably developed, not worn out. And third, my mother bought these for me several Christmases ago. Maybe I needed to gradually wean myself off my couch clothes as part of my full-recuperation process. I believe Dr. Vandoven would agree."

She sat down across from me. "Sure, that's a prescription I'd like to see him write. Let's get him on the phone right now and ask. Here!" She tried to hand me her cell phone.

"It's past office hours, or I'm sure he'd agree."

"Yeah? That you are having deep withdrawal symptoms from shoddy clothes? Is that what this is about?"

"A bit. I may need to go to a meeting tonight for pajamas anonymous," I said, laughing to myself.

"Whatever! Obviously, you're feeling better."

"Whatever? You know how I hate that word. You sound like a teenager. It is such a put-down, without really saying anything." I waved a Kleenex in front of me as a sign of surrender. "Let's go! I'm ready to enjoy a brisk walk and conversation that doesn't come out of an electronic box."

"What? I'm a step above an electronic box?" Diana asked, puzzled.

"No! you're way above the television. You're the good house noise." I watched her face sour. "I love bantering with you. You know that. It's the only part of my day when I feel like I'm winning."

"I'm the good house noise? I know you like to get a rise out of me, but trust me; you are not winning."

"Yeah, that rise of flush and suck of lips is winning!"

We headed out into the cool air of sundown and winter. It was invigorating, though I had to be extremely careful. I watched my feet as they moved ahead of my face. I rubbed my chest along the healing incision. I seemed to be doing that a lot lately.

Walking shouldn't have been emotional, but it was. I felt each muscle flex and release. I discerned each separate beat of my heart and was stirred by the crisp air repeatedly filling my lungs. I focused on blood flow and the chill of canyon breezes, descending from the mountains and raising hair on my neck. We held hands. The sensation of love made the walk light and enjoyable.

I hadn't realized that I walked so slow and deliberately. We were making little progress. I simply enjoyed being out of the house with my favorite person.

Conversation was out of the question. It was too cold to open our mouths. There was enough said by just being with each other and holding hands. Time stretched its arms. We were carefree and cold, though the weather seemed inconsequential. There was a freedom of stride, as I felt my legs stretch into a faster rhythm—faster than before, but still insignificant. The quiet was soothing.

At the end of the driveway, I realized I was gasping for air. My heart was beating like a sledgehammer against my chest. The sound of it inside pulled me out of a wonderful stupor. I glanced back at our house. It seemed hundreds of miles away. My feet walked down two squares of sidewalk, about six more feet. I'm not sure if I had even left my property line. I was beginning to panic, knowing the walk had been very short but feeling as though I had so far to go back.

"I gotta get back. . . . Now! No, let me rest a few minutes." I forced out my breath, stopping mid-stride. I grabbed my chest, taking in air slowly, and sucked in as if it the air was solid. Dread and anxiety filled my eyes.

"You okay?" Diana asked, concerned.

I was trying to catch my breath. Talking was difficult. In slow words, I said, "I'm just having a hard time . . . breathing." I was bent over, gasping for oxygen, as though I had just finished a marathon. Cupping my hands around my mouth, I tried to warm the air as it sifted between fingers. It attacked sharply, like tiny icicles. After staring at Diana for a few long minutes, my breath gradually steadied. "Okay, I'm ready now."

I began walking back. I was a little scared, and the panic in Diana's eyes wasn't helping. I thought I felt better than that. The body seems to recover at its own pace, no matter how strong one's willpower is.

Slowly, we made it back to the porch, through the front door, and up the stairs. I had to stop three times on the way up the stairs for short periods of recuperation. I was irritated at myself and my "stupid heart," as I called it several times during the walk back. I was frustrated, in a sulking, silent way. There is something incredibly defeating about that first push to return to normal. I started out just fine, and then lost it at twenty yards. Not an admirable distance in my mind. I'm sure everyone in their Nike tees and Spandex at Gold's Gym would absolutely laugh. The walk was actually an achievement, but I didn't realize it until much later. *To hell with Gold's Gym.* To hell with elevator recuperation.

Diana held my wrist as we climbed the stairs, concern spread across her face and posture. She spoke in soft tones. I concentrated on my breathing and heart rhythm as I watched my feet lift, slide, and drop. I watched her mouth move. When someone doesn't respond to her, she keeps repeating herself, as though it must be a hearing problem. I looked at her and held my palm up to let her know, politely, to shut up; I was concentrating. She appeared hurt, as her mouth snapped tightly shut and her eyes snapped wide open. She ceased breathing. Her face turned red.

In time, my breathing slowed, my lungs relaxed, and my heartbeat reverted to the offbeat, now normal cadence of a post-cardiac-arrest pulse. What's that saying about how time heals all wounds? It's not just about emotional wounds, though a lot of those accompany the physical scars. My heart may heal, but it will never be 100 percent, and it certainly won't return to the powerful pump of my twenties.

I broke the self-enforced silence as I rounded the top of the stairs and slumped like Jell-O onto my haven, the couch. "Well, that was absurd."

"Give yourself some time. It will happen." Diana crossed her arms and gazed down at my defeated shape.

"No . . . no. I know I need time and all that. I am just plain really not really happy about this STUPID heart and these STUPID lungs. I wanna scream. I want to slap them around. Slap them back into perfection. I don't want a stupid heart and stupid heart heredity." My voice echoed off the walls.

Diana massaged the back of my neck. "I'm not sure what we can do about any of that." She looked a little squeamish, probably because this was a new color for me—the horrid shade of self-pity. "That's why you had the operation. To make your heart better."

I smiled and giggled at myself. "Yeah, the operation was stupid, too."

"Okay, so essentially you're saying everything was stupid?"

"Yes. I had a stupid operation on a stupid heart, and the stupid surgeon used my stupid veins from my stupid legs, and I now I have a stupid recovery."

"Are you done being five years old?" she puffed her cheeks appreciating her own question.

I thought for a minute. "And the stupid walk, to stupid nowhere." I hesitated and raised my eyes to the ceiling. "Okay! I think I'm done. That little tantrum made me feel much better." I was taking full, steady breaths now. The muscles in my arms and legs seemed to have loosened. The indoor air had lost its stale, foul taste. My mood brightened.

"I'm glad—not for the tantrum, but that it's over." Diana smacked me lightly on the shoulder as she giggled, sitting next to me. "What should we do now?"

"How about a stupid dinner?"

"This is going to go on all night, isn't it?"

"Well, yeah . . . stupid."

"I'll go make the stupid dinner. You watch the stupid TV or read a stupid book." She got up to go, shaking her head as she looked at me with raised eyebrows and a mischievous smirk.

"Now you got it," I gave her a thumb's up.

"Yes, but I'm hoping to get rid of it," she said as she disappeared into the kitchen.

Cooking noises began in the next room. I sat and was content to just listen to the sounds of her fixing a meal. Fact it: I was easily entertained.

The next day, after a fairly pleasant night of sleep and a lunch of Campbell's salt- infested chicken noodle soup and crackers, we had visitors. My sister, Annette, and my brother-in- law, Keith, came for a visit, bringing half a dozen of their grandkids and one of their daughters. She had the kids dressed as the Three Wise Men who visited Christ after His birth. Obviously, they had the wrong house. They had on long colorful robes and Arabian headgear. A couple of small hands carried fancy brass containers, supposedly containing frankincense and myrrh. I am sure it was hard to get good frankincense and myrrh in this day and age. I was impressed, and I livened as I studied their faces.

Annette, in the voice of a true pedagogue, told a short story about the birth of Christ, the six (changed by the number of child actors) wise men, and their journey to follow the bright new star to Bethlehem.

Essentially, I received six wise men, though some were young girls. They were all between the ages of three and seven. They looked like sheiks in oversized clothing, straight out of their tents, waiting for their camels to be brought forward for a pleasant, long journey across the desert. My sister and her husband were dressed similarly, with cloth draped over their heads and held in place by fancy colored bands at the forehead. Small blankets were draped over their shoulders, like shawls.

After the story, my sister had the short wise men sing various Christmas songs for me. The children were a bit frightened by the sick, pale guy, but sang beautifully in those high voices only post-toddlers can master. It was incredibly pleasant and extraordinary. For a short time, I needed no medicine for my surgical aches and suture tickles. My breath was relaxed and my position comfortable. The caroling filled my newly commandeered bedroom on the couch. I was tranquil, calmed by the music of tiny voices and lyrics of seasons and memories past. It was a sweet gesture.

Christmas Eve day arrived. The snow was light. The air was calm, and icicles formed a pretty scalloped edge around the soffit of our roof. The branches of trees lining our street were glazed in frozen winter moisture. Tiny drips hung, motionless, from the tips. Our heater cycled more on than off to maintain the thermostat setting. With my blood not pumping as quickly as before, I needed the thermostat turned up. Nothing seemed to get warm. My circulation flowed like a frigid river. I sat cross-legged in front of a heater vent, my deep purple bathrobe forming a chimney, with the flow warming my chest and venting out at my neck. I kept flapping my arms inside the bathrobe to increase circulation. I'm glad no one took pictures. I'm sure I looked ridiculous. But at least I was getting warm.

Kyle had gone with his biological father, a man who visited him a handful of times each year and who separated from Diana shortly after Kyle's premature birth, to his home a couple hours away.

Diana and I were going to my mother's condominium for Christmas Eve dinner. It was one of the traditions of the Huntsman family, not dissimilar to those of other families. Brothers, sisters, kids, too much food, reacquainting conversations, best plates and silverware, token packages wrapped in red Santas and blue snowmen scenes, a trail of smiling porcelain reindeer on Mom's coffee table, a plastic tree with memorable ornaments, end tables decorated with white cotton and tiny cardboard houses, and splashes of red and white figurines everywhere let everyone know how obsessed Mom was with the American Christmas.

The back half of the self-serve table was laden with baked ham with honey glaze, fluffy rolls, real butter on an actual butter plate (no plastic tubs here!), and a salad of mixed greens. Baked beans with chunks of ham and mashed potatoes and gravy filled the front of the table. The savory, sugared smell of sweet-potato pie with cinnamon drifted around the corner from the kitchen as we all stood in a you-first parade before the well-laid-out Christmas serving table.

I was classified as an invalid, being just out of the hospital, so I was graciously placed in front and got to fill my plate first.

Being sick has its rewards. It also has its drawbacks. I really did feel like crap. I was uncomfortable and took breaths through parted lips as if hiking the Himalayas. With each movement, I used my forearm to protect my chest from getting hit or touched, and I carefully kept a distance from others and from objects. My chest was solid, but there's something about having your sternum wired together like a farm fencepost and the flesh of your torso stitched far enough down that you think your pancreas might fall out.

I sat down slowly with my plate, as though the seat cushion was a porcupine and the plate of food a tray of rattlesnakes. *Overly cautious* would not even begin to describe my new-found paranoia. I ate the same way, in tiny, definitive bites, my jaws moving in slow motion. My eyes concentrated on the food in front of me. The conversation at the table was no more than white noise. Diana nudged me a few times, probably to see if I was breathing as she wondered if the insurance payments had been made. I was anxious, dizzy, and nauseous; I ate very little.

I paid minimal attention to the conversation at the dinner table. Knowing my mom, I'm sure she directed it to topics of political incorrectness and shocking innuendo about the government (or anyone associated with an office) or to high-profile news events. She was opinionated and frequently dealt out criticism from her narrow understanding of any truth, past or present. I had been to enough family gatherings to know how the dynamics worked.

She always started out guiding the dinner talk to family stories and events. She congratulated each of us on this, that, or the other. Then, out of nowhere, she slammed a politician or law or religious belief that didn't make sense to her. She was a total sweetheart to her children and friends but had negative opinions on *outsiders*. We nodded and tried to change the subject. Sometimes it worked; sometimes it didn't. It's impossible to argue with someone in their eighties.

My mom came from a different era, one with opinions and prejudices founded in a small mining town with separated areas for people of different heritage. I didn't understand or agree with most of my mom's ideas and viewpoints, but I did love her completely.

After swallowing bits of dinner that wouldn't feed a baby sparrow, I faded away from the table, landed on a stuffed chair, and carefully perched my feet on the matching ottoman. My head was spinning, and my chest heaved as I curled up in a fetal position. I let my face muscles go limp and mumbled every so often as though I was keeping up with the conversation. Prior to my impersonation of an embryo, my energy level had been slightly above zero, but not by much. Laughter and conversation continued. I heard nothing—which was about what I cared to hear. Shortly, I fell asleep.

When I awoke, dinner was over; everyone was sitting on chairs and couches around me. Kyle and Tim asked me if I was okay. I nodded. A few dining room chairs helped with the overflow. My mother wandered around with platters of leftovers and treats, pushing them into everyone's chest with snippets such as, "You can have one more," and "You need to try it," as everyone held one hand up and the other over their stomachs in the universal sign of "full tank." The smell of the feast raised sensations of happiness to my nostrils. The prattling was still at full volume, everyone trying to get a word in, with several conversations going at the same time. I remained sick and lifeless on the white chair.

I feigned sleep when my sisters spotted my half-open eyes and tried to find out if I was all right. Of course, I wasn't all right—hence the curled, lifeless figure in the corner of the room. However, I didn't want to ruin their holiday.

"I'm fine," I muttered defensively to my two sisters. That appeased them. They turned to another conversation.

Diana came over and sat by me. "Can I get you anything?" she said in a low voice, her lips next to my ear.

"Take me home," I muttered. I hoped it was loud enough for her to hear. I thought I was fading into nothingness. I needed to leave before the soft chair sucked me in. I wanted my own house and my own bed—and my own couch.

She came back shortly and squeezed my arm to get my attention. My coat was in her hand. She had to put it on me like she would a child. It would have been humiliating, if I had cared. I didn't. I followed her out like a dog on a leash, nodding my head at everyone as I left. I probably barked out a whimper, but I don't recall. Our two boys followed.

I felt my blood pressure sinking, and I was losing the ability to concentrate. A headache started. The ride seemed to take a long time. I tried to take deep breaths and lay back in the car seat.

We were a few blocks from home when I muttered, "I need to go to the hospital."

Diana's shoulders curled and her breath caught. The boy's eyes widened, and mouths thinned.

I was lethargic and useless. My head spun in both directions simultaneously. I thought my heart was making quivering movements instead of a pumping beat. Tiny chest pains seemed to clamp my throat. I held my hands over my heart, hoping that would make it feel better. My limbs were sore from resting at my Mom's in an awkward position. The heart problem was probably psychosomatic, but my brain was frightened by the possibilities. Once fear takes hold, all reason is shut out.

Now, years later, I assume it was a simple case of angina. Of course, nothing is simple those first weeks after a cardiac arrest. Everything is a big deal. You start to wonder if even a muscle spasm in your foot is related to your heart.

What was odd at the time was that I wanted to see more doctors. I had spent forty-eight years without visiting a hospital and had probably had only three or four doctor appointments since I was six years old. I had always been healthy. Yet, here I was, seeing more doctors in a thirty-two-day period than I had in my entire life. I would have felt pitiful if I hadn't been so sick.

Diana guided me through the emergency entrance. The next thing I remember, I was hooked up to beeping machines and an IV while people in white lab coats stared with concerned faces. Blood was drawn and EKGs were recorded.

Tim were taken to picked up by his mom, and Kyle was taken to Diana's mom's to be watched. It wouldn't be until late that night that I would find out about the boys.

All the applicable tests produced normal results except for a slightly low blood pressure. The results were normal for my heart, that is. My cardiologist had had explained that due to my heart attack and original misdiagnosis, one-third of my cardiac muscle was dead tissue. The other two-thirds of my heart muscle was compensating and gagging in an abnormal, sustainable rhythm. The battery of tests that night in the ER was consistent with those facts. At the time, I was puzzled and concerned that the tests were wrong, or that the staff performing them was incompetent.

There is nothing better than an ER visit to kick up the anxiety barometer. I knew the heart pain I experienced was nowhere near the level of a cardiac arrest, but I was still somewhat new to all this. The ER doctor told me the enzyme count that typically rose after a cardiac episode sometimes takes a while to show. After heavy hydration from ice and water, I began to get comfortable, and my anxiety eased. Diana's face remained helpful throughout. Her eyes told a different story; I saw worry and a hint of fear. It was a stoic attempt, and I loved her for it. It was the blanket of warmth that I needed. I had no healing laughter or smiles—just sweat dripping from my palms and desert dryness in my mouth.

The ER doctor was a young intern. He was diligent and concerned, with insight from phone calls to my cardiologist. He prescribed a "just-in-case" solution of keeping me overnight for observation, even though no adverse signs were found. Diana slept on a chair in my room. She curled into it like content cat. I fell asleep easily, probably through medication, just before the end of Christmas Eve—*Merry flippin' Christmas*.

Sleeping hard, even with the bother of night shift nurses and their probing, I was fully rested when I awoke at seven-thirty the next morning. My spirits were high. I was rejuvenated back to the serrated health I had enjoyed a couple of days prior. It was Christmas Day, but I'm fairly sure I didn't realize it until much later.

Diana looked over at me from one of those half-couch furniture pieces hospitals are famous for. She was trying to stretch her crooked limbs out of the crumbled position she had held while sleeping on a thin-padded, three-foot couch. I wasn't sure when she turned the industrial chair into a couch. Her neck tilted at a thirty-degree angle to her shoulders, her arms pasted to her sides as if they would be of no use for years. She tried to smile at me. It came off more like indigestion. Her hair shot out in all directions. The sympathetic nurse gave her more pity than she gave me.

Dr. Vandoven, my cardiologist, came in after a few short raps of his knuckles on the door. He gave a quick, compassionate look at Diana and walked to my bedside. He said, "All your tests look much better. How are you feeling?" He pushed wires and tubes aside with his hand and sat on the side of the bed.

"I'm ready to go home."

He straightened his back and nodded. "You feel as though whatever episode you had yesterday is over?"

"Completely! It's amazing how a night in the hospital makes one want to recuperate quickly," I lied.

"I understand." The doctor paused, readjusting his rump. His hand rubbed his temple. With a warming grin, he said, "The alternative is more days in the hospital."

"Exactly! Plus, I can't afford the hotel rate."

He chuckled to himself. "There is something to be said for the positive psychological effects of a hospital stay."

We joked back and forth for a bit; he listened to my heart, front and back, had me take deep breaths, and asked about my symptoms. I told him they were minor at the beginning, but fear seemed to have multiplied them. *Maybe it was just too much Christmas. Maybe I should skip all holidays, at least those that aren't cardiac healthy—Halloween, Valentine's Day, Memorial Day.* I mentioned to him that my whole body had felt crappy.

Diana checked me out of the hospital. I felt relieved as I walked to the car by myself and thought about being driven home. I still don't know if the pains were real or part of my internal anxiety. The pulses of those quirky little spasms called angina, real and imaginary, dictate awareness of internal workings I never noticed before—in fact, that I never even knew I had.

I had begun bending and posturing to relieve the spasms associated with angina. There must have been rearranging of internal organs and fibers after the unsettling journey of surgery. My initial response to angina was a panicky state. Finally, I settled into lying to myself that it was nothing. It certainly could have been just a panic attack, as the ER doctor suggested, though it hit like a bull on the rampage. My small movements and a push from positive thinking settled things back into place.

Over the course of a few weeks, I walked as far as I could most days, stopped while resting and regaining lung control, and then walked back to the house in an upright crawl. Eventually making it across the street was a milestone. I celebrated on the other side, breathing heavily. Diana stood next to me, patiently waiting. I was a slow work in progress.

Getting around a whole neighborhood block was another hurdle. It was a process of advancing one driveway at a time. There were days of setbacks, when making it to the next-door neighbor's house was all I could do. Eventually, I made it halfway around the block, at which point the only way back was to turn and keep moving. That first full trek around the block was the best. It felt like a real accomplishment. After that, my walks seemed easier. Recuperation was a slow return to stamina, taking work and time to reach each new gain. There were many proud and memorable moments—I made it to the Anderson home seven houses away, and I was only lightheaded and delirious. It seems so long ago now that it's hard even for me to adequately imagine the frustration.

15

I was walking short distances and feeling pretty good about my progress. An achievement smile kept posting on my face more often than not. I was getting accustomed to the tingling in my legs where my veins were torn out—"harvested," as the doctors called it. *Harvest* sounds as though a farmer and a few migrant workers picked a ripe crop from my calves. It made me wonder if any of the surgical instruments were dark green and made by John Deere. Whatever they called it, it still felt like my veins had been ripped out by the "children of the corn."

My diet changed; I avoided fats and ate fruits and vegetables that had barely graced my kitchen table before. I tossed out one of my main food sources—potato chips. I was still having withdrawals from bags of thin, crunchy, fried oil and potatoes. My mind was consumed by articles and books about heart disease and the things to do to avoid it—uh-oh, too late. Well, at least I could improve my odds of surviving it. I planned to do my best to prevent any more dead heart tissue. I was actually elated by this slow progress to wellness.

Then suddenly things changed again. A whole new malady appeared. I woke up having a hard time breathing. My lungs sort of gurgled as if I was trying to breath underwater—which, essentially, I was. If I remember anything from high school biology, I knew taking in oxygen is critical for life unless you're a plant. I wasn't. For several nights in a row, I was forced to sleep upright, or I couldn't breathe. I was Jacques Cousteau with an empty tank. I would bolt upright, panic, and suck down oxygen like an alcoholic finding a hidden bottle.

Sleeping sitting up was fun and comical as a teenager, traveling in convertibles with wild dreams and crazy friends across state lines. We slept on San Francisco streets lined with look-alike houses in a gold, spray-painted Chevy. I spent nights trying to find a comfortable spot around an enormous steering wheel while fog whitewashed the windshield and cold found entrance through the dashboard and poorly sealed doors. But at forty-eight years of age, sleeping upright, even on a pile of pillows, had lost its entertainment value. I enjoyed my teen years; I just didn't want to re-live them by sleeping upright.

This whole sleeplessness experience was making me cranky. My spine was twisted out of place. My neck creaked and chattered with each tiny movement. One butt cheek was seemingly lower than the other, then they'd switch places, depending on the night. I'm not sure why, but my toes had started to hurt. I would get up in the morning and walk to the bathroom like a contorted old man in a slow-motion seizure, wheezing with each step. My wife thought I was overreacting. Of course, she slept soundly and horizontally.

Each time I laid down flat, I gasped for air. It was the scariest thing I had ever been through. Even slightly elevated, I could not catch my breath. I needed to be at a full sixty-degree angle or more. Being unable to get air in your lungs brings on full-bore anxiety. I cannot imagine what people with emphysema go through. It must be horrid. I'm so grateful that when I tried smoking for a short time in my teens, I didn't find it all that rewarding.

I always thought drowning would be like that. Feeling water enter your lungs and the fright of gasping for air where there is none. Your body needed oxygen, and you would be sucking water into your lungs instead. That first intake of water instead of air must cause immediate panic.

For me, drowning was different. When I was in my early twenties, I ran the rapids of the mighty Colorado River in an eight-man raft. I was never sure why they called it an eight-man raft; it fits only four or five comfortably, with a cooler in the middle and a potato sack of beer on a rope, floating behind. I frequently captained the excursion and took groups of friends along, some experienced, some not.

Most of the runs down the Colorado were relaxed, beer-drinking, sunburned fun. We floated by grazing cows and shot through rapids with exhilaration, all oars in the water. Then we floated lazily through another section of eddies to an area where the water seemed as still as a lake. There was a section between Thompson Bridge and Moab, Utah, that was great for beginners, with just enough rough water to stir things up. That's the area I knew the best. It had Indian petroglyphs, beautiful scenery, and red sand beaches to camp or play on.

One time, a person I took down the river lost his oar to the current. I was the captain of an inflatable raft with three others as my crew, none of whom had ever floated any river before. We were on a seemingly slow part of the river, but the Colorado moves with deliberate herculean force. Without thinking, I jumped in after the oar. I knew better, but the sun and beer had dwindled my brain to a raisin. As happens in rivers, the current pulled me quickly ahead of my friends in the raft. After swimming with the current, I caught up with the oar and grabbed it. I turned to find myself forty yards ahead of the rubber raft. I looked for options. My body hurled further from the others. The water was spring runoff cold; my teeth chattered. I decided to try to swim for shore, which, with an oar in my hand, became impossible. I let go of it, swimming as hard and fast as I could toward the shore.

The current was so strong it kept surging me forward and down the Colorado River. I was quickly overpowered, and my muscles were strained. Totally exhausted, I finally made it to the steep cliff shore. I grabbed at branches and roots of bushes as I swept quickly by. Some tore from my hands, others ripped from the limestone bank. The force of moving water was too strong, and the sparse foliage gave little to grab onto.

I went between two slick rocks and over a small waterfall. In that turbulence I was twisted and pulled down into deep water. Water-soaked debris flicked at my skin. The undertow held me momentarily, then spit me up and out into the rapids. My lungs were crying for air. I was losing the fight to hold my breath. In a panic, I breathed in the muddy water. Instead of the pain I expected, the hazy peace of sleep overtook me as the perfidious force pulled me farther downstream.

Just as everything in me was giving up, I saw a hand above me, slightly illuminated from above. At least, I thought it was above me. I was thoroughly disoriented. With water in my lungs, the sleepy deep beckoning, and air only a couple of feet away, I held both arms up in what I felt was a last effort. The hand from above reached out and grabbed my left wrist, yanking my arm, then swinging me partially into my yellow rubber raft. Another arm grabbed my torso and rolled me further into the safety of the raft. It happened quickly, but my mind took it in as time slowed. I was handled roughly, and my chest was smacked until I finally coughed up the river inside. Air filled my lungs in short, fear-throttled bursts. Again, I coughed up muddy Colorado River water. Another breath of warmed oxygen filled my tremulous body. The coughing and fear subsided. The quivering did not. The terrifying experience felt life-giving and truly miraculous.

I was drowsy and shivering from the bitter temperature of spring runoff. The ninety-degree sunshine did nothing to abate it. Someone wrapped a semi-wet towel around me. Someone else used his body heat against mine to warm me. After time, my breathing slowed, and my shivering became intermittent. I was still cold and scared to death, but grateful to be alive.

In short, I experienced drowning as a sleepy, uncaring situation, a wearing down and giving up. I had taken a breath of water, just as I did air. It was not at all what I had expected.

The sleepless nights were not going away. The extreme efforts to breathe were not going away. I decided to call my cardiologist. He had me come in the next day.

Dr. Vandoven thought I might have pulmonary edema—essentially "water on the lungs." I have little medical knowledge, but even I know I am supposed to have air in my lungs, not water. I know from Biology 101 that I definitely do not have gills.

Apparently, pulmonary edema typically develops when the heart or circulatory system is not functioning properly. Ah—heart attack, heart surgery, it all made sense. If one thing in the human body isn't working well, it affects other parts. I think the opposite is also true. If the heart and lungs are working well, the cells respond, and other parts of the body work better. I wanted this fixed before the rest of my body heard the news and something else went wrong.

Dr. Vandoven set up an appointment with an associate of his in pulmonary medicine. He reassured me that my breathing would return to "stability," and I would have other positive improvements. Hopefully, that improvement involved sleeping horizontally. I was having a tough time walking thirty yards, though, so his reassurances seemed translucent at best. It was like the weather report on the five o'clock news, informative yet meaningless. A look out the window is a better indicator. When the doctor spoke, I heard "sunshine and warm temperatures," but I saw dark clouds forming and wind whipping the trees shortly after. Sunshine may happen later, perhaps even that afternoon. Right then, though, the clouds weren't parting, and I couldn't see the onset of good weather.

My pulmonary specialist was at the same hospital as my cardiologist and my heart surgeon. I felt good about that, though I'm not sure why. It just felt like heart problem home plate or something. The pulmonary doctor looked more like an accountant than a lung specialist. His glasses were the wire rims of the sixties. His hands were large, almost with a swollen look that didn't really fit his body or his friendly, concerned face. They reminded me of the hands of a mobster, made for strangling those with unpaid debt, not made for fixing lungs.

After introductions and the doctor reading my new chart, I was sent with the nurse to another room. She had unimpressive machines with tubes and large, thermometer-looking glassware that she had me breathe into. I pushed the ball up the tube with forced air. I never thought breathing could be so hard, and my efforts to breathe sounded like bad brakes. My lungs felt small and worn out. I repeated it three times. She guided me back to the first room, where I had another wait. Who would have known?

I spent a brief time looking at sunset prints on the walls until the doctor returned. He had me breathe deeply while he pressed his stethoscope against various places on my back and chest. He nodded his head, said I had a fair amount of fluid on my lungs, and quickly scribbled a few prescriptions. He told me one was a diuretic to help me get rid of the excess water, another was an antibiotic for my pericarditis, and the third was something with nitrates that would help something else. I don't remember.

Essentially, I was going to pharmaceutically pee the pulmonary edema out. I asked the doctor about anything orange coming out. He gave me a totally puzzled look and said there were no pigments in the drugs. I gurgled in a breath of relief and let out a slow exhale.

Nothing goes away immediately. I was urinating like a racehorse but still packing pillows and cushions from outdoor furniture onto the bed to elevate my upper body. It's always frustrating when magic pills take their time. I really needed an actual night's sleep, lying flat. Did you know they have reruns of daytime TV programs at three in the morning? I wouldn't waste my time on them during the day, but they seemed engaging in the dark of night.

The extra cushions on our bed worked most of the night. I finally began resting soundly. Then I moved, and the whole house of cards came tumbling down. With bed sheets wrapping my legs in a cocoon, they hung me genuflect, with my neck and head painfully resting face to the carpet. It was such a precarious position that unwinding out of it was a seven-minute struggle. Plus, I had to pee. And I was having angina. And the *Jerry Springer Show* was whispering from the television with two ladies in a cat fight over some ridiculous drama. I was definitely living someone else's life.

Diana mumbled something unintelligible to me—probably "be quiet" or "hold still" or some such endearing, sympathetic phrase. I couldn't see her from my position, but her concern was not helpful. I heard a light snore shortly after her scolding and imagined her relaxed face. My teeth ground together.

Free at last, I ran to the bathroom. This wasn't the first time I had peed through the night, and I assumed it wouldn't be the last. I rebuilt the bedding, pillows, and cushions toward the middle of the bed, carefully pushing Diana to one side. With uneasy stability and precarious balance, I lay atop my creation, trying to sleep in a state between anxiety, rest, and urination, for a few more hours.

There was a side effect from the strong antibiotics. The pills burned a portion of my stomach away, causing me to buckle in half and grimace for several hours after I took each dose. I could eat only soup and drink only water. I began to think maybe the pericarditis was less threatening than the remedy. I quit taking those pills. I called my doctor about the new stomach disorder, and he agreed I should stop taking the antibiotics.

The hole in my middle eventually healed, and I could eat solid foods again. Between the intestinal pain and water breathing, I had slept only about four hours per night. I had also lost weight, and at this point I didn't have a lot to lose.

When the sun streamed through the windows, I was already awake.

After sleeping with my body braced up and my feet downhill for a week, I finally began to take away pillows. After four more days of that, I was down to one large, fluffy pillow; my lungs were being used for oxygen instead of as a fish bowl, and I had received more than my share of diuretic exercise, walking back and forth to pee like a champion. I was going for the gold.

There is an end to each episode of illness. Clinging to the idea of life and the things coming in your future helps a great deal, but medicine and time increases your chances. When these things like an inability to breathe hit, then is the time to hope for the better and know that it probably won't last.

I was able to take my walks a bit more seriously now that I was breathing with both unsaturated lungs, dropping the antibiotics, and finding sleep. I was refreshed as I got up early and enjoyed my fruit and cereal breakfast, sometimes with wheat toast, sometimes without. I became used to one egg per week and a term I had never heard of before—"dry toast." It even began to have flavor and lose its insipidness. I followed heart-healthy diet recipes. Walks became stimulating instead of laborious. I waved at neighbors I had never met at a block away, then two blocks away, then three. Three was my goal. Anything outside that radius didn't exist, unless I was driving a car. I will never be a marathon runner.

I wouldn't have believed it was possible, but driving a car was also a feat. I had this new internal fear that accompanied the prospect of getting behind the wheel. I let Diana drive me everywhere for quite some time, even though I thought I was ready to drive. My mind always ran a short movie clip of the steering wheel crushing my once-open chest that was wired up like a bale of hay as I crashed into oncoming traffic. My smarter self knew this was a ridiculous apprehension, but that didn't make it go away. At these thoughts, I would get tight in the chest and perspire. I could almost feel the twisted metal retainers that held my ribs together loosening, and my chest spreading. I pretended the fear was nonexistent. But it was there with a full-color presentation in the back of my mind whenever I contemplated the task. It was an absurd phobia, I know. I looked it up. I felt a little better about driving after knowing it was a real fear, called *amaxophobia*. It was good to know other people shared the same fear I had surgically inherited.

I waited until I was alone and forced myself into the driver's seat one day. I kept telling my mind how truly silly my fear was. I slipped the key in, turned it, and took a deep breath. The car hummed for several minutes in the driveway. I thought about driving. Images of car wrecks and steering wheels being pried from my body by the Jaws of Life immediately entered my mind, unbidden.

I tried blinking and centering my mind on thoughts of peaceful country roads—perhaps in the French countryside. I put the car in reverse, slowly backing out of the driveway. I was feeling pretty sure of myself. Then I shifted into drive and drove as fast as I could with wheels squealing, dogs barking, and neighbors jumping to the curb. I knew if I was going to do this, it had to be quick. No thinking allowed. The wheels barely held the ground as I rounded street corners. I circled the block once. The car pulled sharply into my driveway as I stomped on the brakes, inches in front of the garage door. Boy, that felt great. I love France.

I waited until my breathing and heartbeat slowed. I got out of the car, smiled, and went in the house to celebrate by sitting on the couch with a tall drink of healthy ice water—Jose Cuervo was out of the question.

As time went on, I began driving to the store and on other short errands. I still held my chest in the car. I could drive, but the anxiety, though much milder, was still there. It is strange; I was more fearful of driving than I was of having bypass surgery. Go figure!

16

January shuffled out the door, and I was looking forward to spring, though I knew winter chilled the ground for at least another month or two. My energy pointed toward getting back to work. My breathing struggled, but I exercised regularly and ate as close to a heart-healthy diet as my lifestyle and taste buds could stand. Angina occurred at times, though putting a nitro tab under my tongue relieved it. I finally understood that climbing stairs at a determined run was bad for me if I wanted to get along with my heart. I realized eating too much sugar raced my heart as much as three cups of espresso used to. Fatty foods made me feel just plain yucky. Goodbye, French fries. Hello, oatmeal.

About this time, I received a refund check from an old insurance policy. The company, it seems, had overcharged me for quite some time. I was elated, reading the amount aloud several times. *Nine thousand, nine hundred, forty-two dollars and twenty-two cents.* Wow! Just in time for a boat to water ski behind.

I perfected my driving skills, concentrated on avoiding the steering wheel smashing into my chest, and drove to a boat dealer I had found on the internet. They had listed a twenty-one-foot Maxum ski boat. It was the boat my bypassed heart and I had decided we both truly needed. During my convalescence, I had studied up on power boats. I had searched the internet for weeks and had looked at boats across the United States. I knew what I wanted. With my new lease on life, I needed to upgrade my old wood boat. The old boat had served me well, but my rebuilt heart needed something with more power and grace. An urgency arose in my mind—my thoughts floated to the necessity.

By the time I pulled into the boat dealer's parking lot, I was out of breath and had developed a high degree of traffic anxiety. Relief washed over me, though, since the steering wheel had not impaled my chest. It was still winter, so unless a boat could break ice, the dealership wasn't selling a lot of them. I was able to park in any one of twenty empty stalls. I turned the car off and walked into the showroom with way too much buyer's anticipation. Perhaps I should have mentioned something to Diana, but now was not the time to quibble.

My head spun as I walked between a twenty-eight-foot boat and a thirty-four-footer. They were grand and shiny and lonely. I had found paradise in rows of fiberglass hulls and gelcoat sheen. The afterlife for me consists of mirror-slick water, a cloudless sky, sun at my back, and a power boat parting the water with grace and agility. The ding from the door when I entered didn't distract hidden salespeople from their coffee mugs and vending-machine cinnamon buns. They apparently didn't want to move until spring. Since I was ignored, I climbed up the ramp between the boats, viewing all of them from a high perch.

I climbed inside the twenty-eight-foot cabin cruiser. The new smell was like an aphrodisiac. I searched below deck and checked out the tiny space for the head, imagining rough water and trying to use the bathroom. There was a cozy bed below deck, the curtains tied back with tiny anchors. The fridge and stove stood shiny and efficiently placed. The table and booth would seat four adults comfortably. The storage was perfect for items that danced in my mind's eye and gave me a boyish grin.

Back up on deck, I admired the navigational gauges and gadgets. I wasn't sure what many of them were, but I was impressed, nonetheless. The captain's chair was soft, comfortable, and commanding. I pictured myself with one hand on the steering wheel and the other holding a glass of wine, with a perfect wake behind me and the sun slowly roasting my back.

Suddenly I heard a voice behind me. "Y'all looking for a boat?"

He had a grin wide enough to prop an eight-foot stud that only salespeople of a certain type can perfect. He readied himself for a possible sale, not knowing he didn't need it with me. At this time of year, I think he was happy to talk to anyone.

"No, not all of us, just me," I responded in a smart-ass, non-caring way. I regretted it as soon as the words came out. I don't mind sarcasm, but rude is another thing.

"What?" he asked.

"Never mind. I'm looking for a boat, but not a motor home like this one. I want more of a water ski boat," I said, deliberately trying to be closer to friendly.

"Oh, okay! What have you looked at?" he asked, scratching the bottom of his ear. He had a tan face and an enormous forehead. I don't mean a bald type of forehead; he had plenty of hair. No, he had a Cro-Magnon-type forehead that stuck out like it had been pumped full of air. A golf ball nose rested below his forehead, and traces of ancient acne scarred his flat cheeks. His chin seemed unfinished, as though his neck started immediately below his smile.

Being around salespeople all my life, I am always suspicious. I see through their tactics and read them quite well. Years of training salespeople have given me an edge. His smile threw me off guard. It was warm and natural. There was honesty in his eyes. It felt good to talk to him. This man had natural warmth. Without many words exchanged, I knew he liked people.

I looked back at the boat. "Actually, I saw an ad on your website for a twenty-one-foot open bow."

"That one is right down there." He pointed to his right. "That's a heck of a buy."

I wondered if he would have said the identical words about the one I was standing on if I said that's what I was looking for. I followed him down the ramp and stairs. He made small talk about work, wife, children, where I lived, and boating vacations as we proceeded to the boat. I thought I wanted. Small talk is innocuous and numbing, but we all do it. It seems to come quickly and unknowingly, right after the greeting of, "Hello, what high school did you attend?" It is a rattle of a few questions and answers that spurt out, almost from subconscious thought. It is a reflex.

I've always wondered why silence is such a hard animal to hold comfortably for long. I feel at ease with Diana. We have reached that plateau of understanding where a fine dinner without verbal conversation is comfortable. We communicate with head nods, eye glances, a tip of our glasses, a raise of an eyebrow, a slight change of posture, and tiny hand gestures. Oh, we talk outright a lot, about every subject in the universe. We enjoy playfully joking about pleasant as well as unpleasant topics, and we love bickering and religious debates. In fact, we probably talk more than most couples. But the silences are also truly enjoyable.

I blocked out the salesman's voice until we got to the boat in the online ad. "This is the twenty-one-foot V-hull," he said.

It looked great. It wasn't ostentatious, like the twenty-eight-foot boat. It was a perfect boat for my family and, of course, for me. Excitement bubbled through my sewn-up chest. I tried to hold my emotions steady, showing little interest, while my mind was jumping up and down. "Looks good," I said nonchalantly. I didn't want to appear too ready to buy. I wanted *the deal*, but he needed to work for his commission.

The V-hull was maroon with white above the water line and a deep maroon topside. I strolled around it, spying for nonexistent imperfections and scratches. The gel coat finish had been waxed and was gleaming off the fluorescents. I walked up the wooded stairs and boarded her. Everything was shined and polished to showcase perfection, of course. The white seats were well padded with plenty of storage beneath the cushions. It smelled of vinyl polish rubs and boat wax. The salesman told me this was a trade-in with very few hours on it. He rambled on while I nodded now and then but mostly ignored him, engrossed in admiring "my" boat.

My mind had gained full ownership the moment I sat in the tuck-and-rolled white captain's seat. It fit contentedly on my back and rump. The gauges dazzled me as I held the steering wheel firmly at ten and two. I had no fear of *this* steering wheel. The salesman showed me how the seat adjusted. It was already pre-set for me, so I just nodded at him. I think he knew he had me when I didn't leave the seat for five minutes. I touched gauges and looked in the glove box, or whatever one calls it on a boat. Gravity held me firmly in the captain's chair. Finally, I stood up slowly and moved away.

In this boat, my breathing was evenly paced. I felt content and healthy. Angina was somewhere far away, on a distant shoreline where the sun never set.

I asked the salesman his name again. It was Burl. *Well, that didn't fit. He looked more like a Thomas or a Fredrick, but definitely not a Burl. Isn't a* burl *an outgrowth or something on a log?*

I worked Burl over on the price. When I thought I had the right deal, I told him fine, but I needed him to store it here until spring, without charge. Apparently, that was not a problem.

I bought it on the spot that day. They would de-winterize it and put in a new battery when I picked it up. I never even heard the motor run. I didn't care. I was still feeling the bow lifting over each wave with water splashing off the sides.

I drove home full of energy and smiles. As I turned the key off on my truck, a thought hit me deep in my head. I needed to tell Diana we had just purchased an incredible, open-hull, two-hundred-and-sixty-horsepower boat, full of fun, sun, and adventure. I wasn't sure her enthusiasm would be the same as mine. I could envision her face contorting. I was pretty sure it wouldn't be one of those sacred, silent times we sometimes enjoy. It might involve loud voices and finger pointing. Perhaps I should wait until it was time to take the boat out of storage, in the spring, to share this gift I had bought for "us."

This whole thought process was tearing apart my exhilaration over the project. It made me feel better to name it. I called the boat my "Exhilaration Project." I was hoping it would catch on among the other adult members of our family, namely Diana. I gained more enthusiasm as I thought about all the family boating adventures we would have. The memories alone would be golden. I was already lining them up and using the acronym EP to solidify the whole fantasy.

I thought about leaving a message on Diana's phone about the "Exhilaration Project." I decided against it. That would allow hours for her pot to build up steam.

That evening I gave her the news. At first, she appeared to be just fine with the whole buying-a-boat-without-your-spouse's-approval idea. (I held on to my backup: "Remember, I just had a cardiac arrest.") Then she calmly came up with a frightening wrinkle. She thought we should "level the playing field, so to speak." I had bought a boat without consulting her; she could hit the stores tomorrow and pick up ten to fifteen thousand in clothing and jewelry. She said something about needing to enjoy some of the fun I had enjoyed today.

"Surely that would be copacetic, right?" It wasn't really a question. She added, "Apparently, that's how marriage works. I should be able to go on a shopping spree without any hint of consideration for my husband, right?" She made the word *husband* sound like an expletive. She was using that snotty, little voice thing she does, too. I hated that.

I feigned heart problems. I grabbed my chest and began breathing slowly with gasping breaths. I leaned forward, looking at the floor, my face contorted in agony. I mumbled something about doing things for the family. I kept one eye on her. She scowled. Okay, so I know I'm not perfect. I knew it was a pathetic try. I began to laugh out loud at myself and her.

"You think a heart attack is going to make me change my mind?" she said, her face red. I glanced up enough to see her clenched fists. I could tell this church-going love of my life wanted to slug me, so I lowered my head again. She patted me on the back, saying sarcastically, "You just keep thinking this is okay!"

"You don't seem very excited about the boat I bought us. Maybe you don't understand the family exhilaration thing." I emphasized the word *family* as I kept my head bowed. I thought I might need to protect my face.

"Oh! I'm excited, all right . . . not the way you're thinking, but I'm very, very, very excited." Her teeth were making a grinding sound. Her arms were folded hard. Her breath seemed to pound down in wet bursts upon my head. I knew she was going to become didactic. I had been through this before. After so many years of marriage, we know each other so well; we can finish sentences and anticipate responses. The problem is that both of us have that extra sense. I heard the lecture in my mind before she opened her mouth.

"Did you really believe I would be happy about my husband spending large sums of money on a new boat without talking to me? You just got out of cardiac surgery. You can barely drive a car. You breathe like you just finished a marathon. You are afraid of anyone touching your chest or even getting too close to it. Do you really think this is the time to buy a boat?" She was on a roll.

I knew her questions were rhetorical, but I needed to slow down their progress. "But, I thought—"

Her index finger interrupted me. I was better off keeping quiet. I held my chest for my own comfort and her sympathy. I wasn't receiving much of either.

"You bought a boat without consulting me."

"Well technic—"

"You really want to interrupt me right now?"

Like a naughty child, I shook my head. My bottom lip stretched over the top one, holding it tight to my teeth. I don't always know when to keep quiet. I would try now.

"In your mind, you actually think it was okay to buy this expensive toy for yourself?" she asked, every word laced with sarcasm.

I looked up to answer. I wanted to talk about the "Exhilaration Project," but she wasn't having any of that right then. Her finger came up again. I said nothing. I gazed at her with as much innocence as my face could hold—mouth tight as a locked door.

"You bought a boat. I know you mentioned a boat you liked the other day. I thought you were just trying to keep busy. I didn't think you would go out and buy . . ." Her anger was searching for a word, "the damn thing. I really have to . . . something. I don't even know what." She began pacing.

"And what about this check you received? When did that come?"

My eyes hit hers. I was thinking *uh-oh*.

"You can answer now."

I cleared my throat and readjusted myself on the couch. "It . . . uhhhhh . . . it came yesterday."

"I don't believe you mentioned it to me yesterday."

"I'm on a lot of medication," I said, as though that was a perfectly good explanation.

"Medication, huh! You may need a lot more if I decide to pummel you."

"Go ahead. I deserve it." I held my arms up as if blocking a right hook.

"Don't tempt me." The beginning of a smile formed on her lips. Her eyes softened.

We batted the discussion back and forth for an hour or more. After a while, our voices lost their edge. It was no longer a one-way conversation. We listened. We tossed slightly biting comments. We laughed. I asked for forgiveness; she smacked my arm once or twice.

After a few hours of internal family therapy, Diana asked, "Why do I love you so much?"

"Because I'm full of surprises," I responded.

"One more surprise like this, and I'll surprise you with papers I know how to write, professionally." Her threat was half-hearted. After a time, the tightness of the muscles around her mouth and eyes became slack. The crow's feet disappeared. Something had softened her.

"Do you want to see the boat?" I asked, hopefully.

"I assume they are closed."

"No . . . no, I have a picture of it from the internet," I responded.

"That would probably make my day," She said with a sarcastic tone, then a pause. "It would be thrilling to see a fifteen-thousand-dollar picture of what you spent 'our' money on."

"It was an incredible buy. It is in perfect condition, almost immaculate. In a couple of months, it will sell for ten thousand dollars more. No scratches, pristine seats, and upholstery, barely a hundred hours on the motor. They signed a statement that the engine runs perfectly. When we pick it up, they'll put the prop in a bucket, and we can watch the motor start right up. It has the power to glide swiftly across the water. Your hair blowing in the breeze. Can you picture that in your mind? Can you feel the wind whisking your hair back and the sun on your face?"

"Are you working on a car lot here?" The question came through her teeth with a half-smile; she was thawing a little. "And by the way," she went on, "I had my hair blowing in the breeze—let me rephrase that, blowing in the *wind*—before. Remember when we first met, and you had that shiny, red convertible? I recall the blowing part. I didn't much care for it. I would get all decked out for a date and you would re-dry my perfect hairdo into something simulating Medusa."

"Medusa had snakes. Boating is all about freedom, waterskiing, fresh air, and gliding with nature."

"Whatever!" Her arms were folded in front of her chest, again. Her posture was as rigid as steel, again.

I tried another angle. "You know you love going in our wooden boat." I knew as soon as I said it that was the wrong approach. I should have grabbed my chest and played the heart attack card again.

She gained a whole new emphasis and fervor. "Oh, yeah! What about the other boat? The Father's Day boat Kyle and I bought for you? Is this new one mine and the old one yours? Hmm . . . maybe I just got a new boat."

We had a nineteen-foot wood boat with a fifty-horsepower Evinrude in the back yard. At one time, it was my prize possession. Diana bought it for me at a garage sale. She paid a hundred dollars. Actually, Kyle kicked in twenty-five of his hard-earned, lawn-mowing money, and she paid the rest.

I spent a month sanding and recoating the wood hull. The old seats had been coated in the look of a 1950s yellow kitchen chair. Diana re-upholstered the seats in a new maroon vinyl. The boat had a wild-dog look when we first brought it home. A lot of elbow grease, fiberglass, new cables, gel coats, and polish later, it became a viable, stylish boat. It also didn't have a motor, so my hundred-dollar boat cost me another thousand plus change for a used motor, new battery, and a hundred other little things. It did come with four Mae West lifejackets from the fifties. Except for softening the seat, the lifejackets were useless. The trailer was adequate, especially after I ground off the rust and applied a coat of black paint.

After I finished all the work on the deep v-hull boat, we took it to a lake and backed it down the ramp into waveless, blue water for its maiden run. I turned the key; it started right up, just like it had in my back yard. I was all grins and tingles as we loaded our family in and motored out into the lake. It turned left with perfect grace. I tried to turn right. Nothing happened. It would only go straight or left. I tried turning it again and again, still, it wouldn't head toward the right.

Frustrated and filled with expletives I kept to myself, I let off on the gas and checked it out while it bobbed in other people's wakes. A small metal part I made for the steering kept it from maneuvering to the right. It was too long, and I had no way of fixing it in the water.

We motored around the lake, doing concentric circles to the left. We had fun laced with frustration. The kids laughed at my boat, circling around and around. We thought of naming it "The Lame Duck." After the trip, I fixed the steering. We had a lot of fun and memories in that boat, but it was time for a new one.

I was quickly losing control of the conversation. "I thought we would sell my old boat and put the money into my new one."

Her posture was still stiff. "Your new boat?"

"Well, yeah! I know I didn't talk to you about it, but I did buy it with extra money I received."

"Oh, I had this absurd notion we were married. Yours is mine and mine is yours." There was a fringe of laughter in her voice.

We kid around with each other so much that I wasn't completely sure if she had lightened up or was still irritated. I tried the teasing approach, since it's my nature. "But honey, you got the hardwood floor in the kitchen."

Her arms uncrossed. "So, is it only the hardwood floor, or do I get the dishwasher and the cabinets? Perhaps a set of glassware? What else is mine?"

"Sure, you can have the whole damn kitchen, as long as I can borrow a spatula and a frying pan once in a while."

Seriousness came over her. "Okay, I've had enough with all the crap. You really feel good about this boat?"

"Incredibly good!" I responded eagerly. There was a sense she was trying to understand. "I see it as a sign of getting better and water skiing and summers together. It's something we need as a family."

Diana is a wonderful fit for me and me for her. Where I fall down, she rises up, and vice versa. I have more voids that she fills than she has for me to cover. But we work well together. It's not that we agree on everything; that's hardly the case. But we talk things out and manage to hold our relationship together. I think it has something to do with respect and insanity. We generally know when to concede and when to debate. We are as close as a couple can be and still retain their autonomy.

"Well, all kidding aside, I hope it's a wonderful thing, this out-of-the-blue possession. It was a bit on the crazy, spontaneous side. But, fine. You realize you owe me big time, right?" she asked sharply as I nodded vigorously. "You bought a boat in the middle of winter? I'm trying to get behind the heart patient insanity." After a short pause, "It may take me a while."

"Oh, thank you for understanding a delusional man, but it was the right thing to do. You'll get it this summer at Lake Powell."

"Yeah, just don't get cocky and think this will work any other time."

We embraced, her head shaking in exasperation and me rocking my head up and down in earnest agreement.

17

Over the next couple of months, I continued traversing the stepping-stones of recuperation. I began eating more and healthier. My pallor—from an ancestry of Vikings and Welshmen—was returning. The morning and evening doses of prescription pills had fewer repercussions, as my body quit asking, "What the hell's that?" I no longer took one pill at a time. I had built it up to a small handful, like three pills. My outside walks were less nauseating and painful. I had regained my posture. My anxiety from body murmurs was subsiding. My positive attitude returned—first in short bursts, then in rapid fire succession. My visitors lost that expression on their faces that said they were envisioning me surrounded by a ridiculous abundance of flowers, lying in a pine coffin on a mound, with winter-dead gray trees and overcast skies. I was close to normal.

I still held my chest unnecessarily and often. I usually did it while laughing at jokes or when sitting close to steering wheels. The couch was getting less wear and tear. The pillows had been put away. The TV remote batteries were dead, and I didn't care. The pericarditis and pulmonary edema had cleared up, leaving me far from gurgling with each breath. I slept only at night and lying flat, on a single pillow. I was reading voraciously again, about three or four books a week. I considered having sex more frequently and lost the fear of my heart short-circuiting during such events. From time to time, I made dinner for Diana, though I could have held out a bit longer. I was being pampered less but working on a relapse to stretch it out—though I was pretty sure at this point that Diana wouldn't fall for it. My body wasn't 100 percent, but I was really enjoying the tangible health change from a few months earlier. I was scheduled to be back to work in a few days.

I still had one annoyance: the sore leg from the surgeon removing my saphenous veins to attach to my heart. It still bothered me that they call it *harvesting*. That sounds too sci-fi. The pain and numbness hadn't gone away. The prognosis was that it could last a couple of years or more. These are the things one finds out much later, as the brain and leg muscles begin wondering why they yanked the veins out and where they put them.

I was told when the saphenous vein is removed from your leg, the blood flow is simply rerouted. My surgeon, Dr. Thorn, explained it as like a traffic detour on city roads.

My mind, of course, pictured it as a road ending with a flashing-arrow traffic sign, with all the drivers confused as they start funneling down smaller side roads. I saw dug-up asphalt, barricades with those blinking yellow lights, and men wearing orange vests, leaning on shovels and telling dirty jokes. I imagined dirt mounds in the road that looked freshly dug but permanent, while the traffic stopped for extended periods, trying to find a way around. Bumpers attached to other bumpers and movement was sluggish, going forward in one-foot increments. The heat and smog from the cars was making everyone's travel just that much more miserable. With luck, by noon the next day the cars would make it to their destinations. In other words, his traffic comparison did not sound all that promising.

I tried explaining it back to Dr. Thorn. "So, my blood is going to come to this detour. It is going to back up and flood areas inside my leg while looking for an alternate route. I assume the other detours are not as big as the original ones you're removing. Right? Are you sure this is the best plan?"

My pompous surgeon had looked at me the way one glances at a lamp or a wood chair in the corner. He went on to explain the other parts of the procedure. It was apparently a didactic lecture, not a conversation. No questions were to be asked, or he would answer only the queries he deemed worthy. I guess he never subscribed to the saying, "There are no dumb questions."

After surgery, I ended up with those white, three-inch, wormlike scars on the inside of my left leg. I have five of them. They were points of numbness and irritation for years. They remind your body that when "harvesting" good veins, the legs rebel and are annoyed for quite some time. On the positive side, it was convenient for my heart to have spare parts only a couple of feet away (no pun intended).

Vein excavation pain is one of the things the doctors don't prepare you for. Getting the heart fixed is priority, as it should be. The details can be addressed later—but later, those details seem really important. Or maybe they tell you, but you don't listen due to the shock of impending heart surgery. The impact of simple problems is lost as a result of other thoughts, like survival.

Another post-procedure dilemma I don't remember being told about was the chest tubes. Waking up from surgery with new plastic appendages growing out of your torso, draining fluids you're not sure you want anyone to see, is debilitating and frightening. I know for a fact I wasn't told about those when I went in to surgery. I was afraid to touch them. They reminded me of the clear gas hoses on the lawnmower. The correlation was upsetting. They called them drainage tubes, but I couldn't help wondering if things from the outside were getting inside, too.

The nurse explained that they would be removed, shortly, whatever time frame that might be, and the holes would seal up. Her explanation didn't help. It was bad enough that there were IVs and hundreds of feet of tubes and wires attached to most of my surface area, but drainage tubes? And they were an intimidating large diameter, more pipes than tubes, one more thing that made it hard to fall asleep. Thank goodness for the sedatives and surgical exhaustion that lured my mind away from the reality of hospitalization and the recovery room.

During the months after my surgery, I was recuperating nicely, though at the time small advances seemed completely inconsequential and inadequate. I wanted a quick recovery. But looking for one was like trying to find an open restaurant for lunch in a small town on a holiday. They are not going to be open. If you wait around long enough, one will finally flip its sign over and heat up the grills—but it will probably be in a day or two.

I am not a patient person. Never have been, never will be. I expect immediate gratification, but I grudgingly accept reality. It is a hard task to do both.

I was doing two days per week at the Cardiac Therapy Gym at the hospital. They had me do the treadmill until dizziness, gasping lungs, and my heart beating in eruptions outside my chest took over. Then they would say, "Okay, that's enough." I always felt like those old cartoons of lovesick ducks and coyotes with their hearts pounding through their chests, only without the love. The physical therapists called it "improvement therapy." I told them it was sadistic manipulation.

Before my heart was remodeled, I don't remember having any trouble running a treadmill or climbing a mountain. Now, the therapist put me on an upside-down bike machine, making me pedal it with my hands and arm muscles until blue veins were popping out of my forehead. My arms maintained the impression of pedaling for several minutes after I walked away from the machine. A time or two, I swear my arms were still rotating as I walked out of the hospital gym, like some geriatric loony.

After a few weeks of their torment, I was told my insurance wouldn't pay for any more sessions. I would have to pay $120 each time out of my own pocket. I opted to save the money and torture myself with faster walks in my neighborhood. That was one expensive gym. I could go to Gold's Gym for about ten dollars a month and save $120 per session after the first day.

Fortunately, I'm not one who gets embarrassed when treadmilling on a level speed of two point two when all the other treadmillers are set at six and run like the wind. It may take me a bit longer to move the belt a mile, but my compadres down the line are still pre-heart-attack patients. With all their French fries and soft drinks, they'll catch up to me soon enough.

18

Thinking back . . . Hell stormed into our life in the year 2000. The stable girders of our world turned to sun-rotted plastic, cracking, snapping, leaving jagged edges and crumbling down on top of us in shards of emotional and physical debility. It was devoid of "the best of times" and busting over with "the worst of times."

The year 2000 was the beginning of many life-changing events, spaced out just enough to let us barely catch our breath before we were pushed over the cliff by yet something else. Everyone has those periods of lows, where one bad thing follows another. It was our turn. We had been given too many obstacles, too big, too soon. Toward the end of the year, one was my heart attack and subsequent surgery. I'll share a bit about the others now.

New Year's Eve of 1999 appeared to be good. Diana and I were heading into a new year with potential and grace. We made excellent resolutions, all with great intentions, as in previous years. Both of us were holding firm to our short list of ideals—be kind, finish certain projects, limit television—with seemingly doable aspirations. We used the first few weeks into the year, working toward those attainable goals, knowing full well that life would happen. Time and stamina would wear down those lists until they would be thought of as next year's resolutions. Then they would become merely an idea, a breeze that had passed and blown over the mountains, never to return again. The printed pages would get lost among paid bills, magazine articles, and recipes cut out for future consideration. It was a cycle we had followed before.

There was a lot of mystery, anticipation, and anxiety leading up to the year 2000. It was the year of Y2K. It was the year computers were supposed to stop working because of their internal clocks. Chaos was to ensue. Public transportation would cease to function. People would be stranded everywhere. The government would fall apart as computers ceased their everyday functioning. All clocks would cease their numbered cycle. Airplanes would stop in midair. Trains would bunch up in stations across America, France, Italy. and all the countries of the earth. It was to be catastrophic.

I was supposed to fly to Las Vegas for the yearly electronics show, but my boss was so concerned about Y2K shutting down all electronic clocks that he cancelled my flight. He decided instead that we would take his van and drive the six hours to Vegas (as opposed to taking a forty-eight-minute flight). Six hours of snow-packed roads sounded absurd to me and not all that much safer than flying through Y2K. Also, I had ridden with my boss before. He drove at the marked speed plus thirty mph, and tailgating was ritualistic to him, like a never-ending prayer to clear the path. His habit was to follow the preceding car, leaving barely enough space between their back bumper and our front for a ream of paper. He continued this until the vehicle in front of us finally moved out of *his* lane. For him, driving was more of a competitive game than a mode of transportation. I really didn't want to play in his game. I was more worried about riding in his van than anything Y2K could throw at me.

The world hadn't fallen apart during the first month of Y2K. There weren't any airplanes dropping from the sky. My computer worked, as did everyone else's. The internet was still intact. The electronics around the world did not implode. The year 2000 began the same as 1999.

On February 4, 2000, my birthday grabbed me, threw a dinner in my honor, and tossed a few returnable and fewer almost useful gifts my way. The country was still worried about Y2K, but still nothing happened. I blew out candles flaming on top of a pumpkin pie (my wife knows I don't really like cake), then the day passed by at a gallop, leaving me one year older. The next day, I felt little difference between the age of forty-seven and forty-eight. I wasn't any taller or smarter, but I was having a harder time keeping thin—except for my hair.

In contrast, the previously meaningless date of February 7 was life-altering for both me and Diana. Neither of us was prepared or could have been prepared for what it brought.

February 7 that year was before my heart attack, so the worst thing in my day-to-day life was trying to find the car keys in the morning. Of course, stubbing my toe was a close second. There was order to my life. It had its highs and lows, but they were small bumps, inconsequential dips, and occasional beautiful vistas.

The seventh of February was a quiet morning. Then my cell phone rang. It was Diana, spewing out completely nonsensical information in a wild, hurried babble. It took me several seconds to piece together the verbal puzzle she was throwing my way. Kyle, our thirteen-year-old son, had a gran mal seizure on the kitchen floor. They were now at his doctor's clinic. My eyes quit blinking and my lungs stilled. She was taking him to the emergency room at Primary Children's Hospital. She would call me from there after she knew more.

I hung up. Emptiness surrounded me. I stood up and then sat back down. I wasn't sure what to do. Kyle had always been healthy and ingenious at solving mechanical problems. He was a friend to everyone and excellent in school. *A seizure!* He must be scared to death. And Diana, how is she handling this? My mind was racing all over the place. After several incoherent minutes, I told my secretary I was heading to Primary Children's Hospital to find out what was happening to Kyle. I explained very little but enough that she hurried me out the door.

I had seen Ed, a friend at work, have seizures. I had also watched a few people in the hospital where I worked during college have them. I knew what the uncontrollable tremors looked like. I knew about the terrible headaches afterwards. I recalled Ed sliding down the rough wall as his body fell limp just before he passed out and then trembled on the ground. I remembered the look on Ed's face just before a seizure started. He had had years of seizures and knew what was happening, and it still took him by surprise. This had never happened to Kyle before, and he wouldn't even know what hit him. It would be terrifying for him to lose control like that. I wished I had been there and that I understood seizures better. And I wondered where the seizure had suddenly come from.

As is often the case when worry overrides everything, I messed up and went to the wrong hospital. I arrived at the old Utah State Children's Hospital. It had been bought and reconstructed as a Shriner's Hospital. Contractors were still working on several sections of the old red brick building. Scaffolding embraced the side where I pulled up. Large cranes on two sides of the hospital gave it a prehistoric look. I parked in front, trying to understand where I was.

A light went on and my brain let out an expletive. I remembered the new Primary Children's Hospital and where it was located. I closed my eyes and pictured the right hospital, gray and turquoise with bands of windows and futuristic architecture. I was several miles away. I took off, my ears heightening to the sound of the road speeding under my tires, almost hitting a worker pushing a wheelbarrow of dust and sheetrock.

I maneuvered the narrow avenue roads quickly and without any roof-mounted lights pressing me to pull over. My God was with me. The restrictive signs along the way were not. With speed, anxiety, and tire noises, I made it to the right place and was out the door almost before my truck settled into park.

I found the emergency entrance with a red blinking light above the sign. I stormed through the doors like a madman. Kyle and Diana huddled in a corner, sharing a children's book. It all looked so natural and normal. They appeared comfortable—no seizure. I'm not sure what I expected, but this calm scene in the waiting room was not it. I wanted the staff to have them in a room, examining him and finding answers. Kyle's pale, worried face glanced up. Diana seemed catatonic but feigned a smile that disappeared quickly. The three of us embraced. Damn emergency rooms.

Emergency always means hurry and get here, then wait until we can get to you. It should state that on the door. My emergency is not theirs. Thirty minutes had passed. Diana had not yet been called in to see a physician. Time was slowing down and our patience was grinding to a halt. I looked over the group of patients-to-be. One young boy's elbow was dripping blood. Another child sobbed in her mother's arms in fits, her cries fluctuating like a swinging gate. Still another little girl had a purple rash that snaked up her neck and branched out in reddish fingers along one cheek. All these children had ghastly, foul things happening to their small, innocent bodies.

I paced back and forth for a minute or two. That didn't help, so I went to the front desk to find out how much longer it would be. They seemed to know less than I, but at least they were rude about it. The receptionist gave me that inhale and eye movement of annoyance. It seemed we were not the only people waiting, and they would get to us in a "timely" fashion. I started to wonder if I would be blowing out my next birthday candles in the ER.

I tried sitting in those chairs that had held so much youthful pain. My comfort zone was somewhere between falling on cacti and drifting in a foul pond of green muck and dead fish. Diana and I sat, shifting rump positions in sync with each other. Sweaty palms held tight together. These was nothing to say.

Suddenly Kyle's eyes glazed over and rolled back. He dropped forward and began trembling uncontrollably on his chair. His arms and legs quaked and flung in every direction. His back arched, teeth clenched, and body spasmed as we held on to him as if we knew what the hell to do. I yelled profanities along with the word *Help!*; in response, the receptionist pushed buttons and made phone calls with calculated efficiency. I'm not sure if it was the loud *HELP* echoing through the emergency room or the expletives before and after that caused her to react. Whichever, she gained clerical momentum from her previously inert mass. Amazingly, she did more than sit and scowl.

Nurses and doctors sped down the sterile, white hallway. Diana comforted Kyle, though he had no idea she was there, as his tremulous body still quaked on the floor. I knelt by Kyle then waved at the approaching gaggle of white and blue, as if I were having my own episode. A stretcher pushed me out of the way, and Kyle was lifted and wheeled to a room for immediate attention.

That attention was the highlight of our day.

We followed Kyle's stretcher to an oak door. A palm was sternly shoved in front of our faces with a command to wait where we were. An air of emptiness and abandonment drifted over us. The impenetrable thickness dissolved into alarm and anxiety as we bobbed our heads like freed Jack-in-the-boxes at the six-by-eight-inch window. All we could see were gauzy curtains and white jackets on people who were scuffling around. The whole scene was surreal. This couldn't be happening to us. It was too graphic and substantive. Kyle's life was being turned upside down, and he was taking us with him. Diana and I started sentences that faded off into babbling prattle. Our stomachs twisted and growled as we held our carpeted ground in front of the wood door.

I couldn't figure out what to do with my hands. I was constantly repositioning them. I folded my arms with my hands in my armpits, then my fingers locked behind me, then I shoved my hands in my pockets, then my hands were tightly grasped at my side, then they were in a praying position as scattered thoughts swirled through my mind. Eventually, as though both of us danced to the same dismay, I caressed my wife's back as she clung to my waist. We held that stance of needing each other for what felt like the better part of forever.

Diana and I paced the hall without leaving sight of the door with our hands interlocked, wearing matching looks of tight-throated soberness. As we heard phantom sounds from the door, anticipation cranked the muscles in our necks. The false alarm noises, both real and imagined, were as deafening as the silence. We memorized the carpet and the brush strokes layered on the two pictures hanging down our hall. Our eyes scanned imperfections of maintenance—wall gouges and a burned-out florescent bulb—as we paced.

Life took its time. Hours and hours passed.

After what seemed like forever, a petite lady doctor came down the hall with critical-care-news splashed across her face and broadcast in her deliberate stride. We knew she was coming toward us, even though she hadn't come through the door we were guarding. We walked toward her. She stopped a pace away and introduced herself as Dr. Lynn Bryson. Handshaking etiquette relieved some of the tension. The hallway had become quite busy; we had been blindly oblivious to it. With a wave of her finger, Dr. Bryson led us down our hall into a room around a corner, virgin territory.

Her shoulder-length hair bounced when she rounded the corner. She was a small package with an air of physician's lineage, tenderness, and vast knowledge behind a crinkled forehead. Her greenish-gray eyes sparkled behind a trace of makeup. Her neck was slight and dainty. She walked with determination. We struggled to keep pace with her.

In this quiet room, Dr. Bryson explained the process used to determine Kyle's malady. At first, she spoke to us as if we both held My Little Ponies to our chests. In time, her voice lowered, and she began using the vocabulary she was schooled in. The blood work, the exam, and the CT scan were laid out, leading us toward being informed but giving no clue yet about where we were going. We talked about his two seizures. She asked if there had been any prior hints of a physical or mental problem. Diana explained that he was smart in school and usually did well but seemed to have trouble with math lately. He had been tested for that, and there was another test scheduled for that Friday. In general, though, Kyle was strong, healthy, and intelligent. There were a lot of questions and few answers.

The day was a whole new adventure disguised as a nightmare.

The news Dr. Bryson laid out was life-altering. From preliminary tests, we were told Kyle had a brain tumor. The doctors hoped it was surgically treatable, but it would take several days before we would know. The next step was for Dr. Bryson to perform a biopsy. Somehow, she made drilling a hole into our son's head and inserting instruments to remove tumorous matter from his brain sound as simple as picking up a loaf of bread from a convenience store. It would be a touch more expensive, of course, though we didn't think of that at the time.

The CT scan showed the tumor, which she lit up on a screen in front us. Dr. Bryson had to point out the difference between healthy tissue and diseased cells of something—perhaps cancer. Once we knew what we were looking at, the mass centered in his brain appeared to be a vile, health-sucking octopus. We were told Kyle's biopsy was scheduled for the next morning. Our hand-hold tightened. We both stared at the floor.

We arrived at Kyle's hospital bed in intensive care. Pull curtains separated him from a roomful of children hooked up to imposing machines that pumped and quacked and buzzed. All this childhood disrupted was strung with a depressing overcast of who would live and who would die. He was settled in and medicated enough to be only slightly coherent. He conked out as we talked to him about tomorrow's surgery. Our chests were so heavy laden with anxiety that breathing seemed unnecessary and impossible.

Nurses were kept busy, going from small patient to small patient in repetitive waves. When it was Kyle's turn, they checked his monitors and looked him over for tell-tale signs of both good and bad. Then they flashed us a gracious smile moved on.

A nurse procured a room where we could stay the night. The parent rooms at the hospital were slightly smaller than a small-town jail cell. Ours had a bed; a few curled, fake-brass coat hangers screwed to the wall; a runt corner shelf; and twelve inches of floor to slide in and out. It was perfect.

I was exhausted and slept for a few hours, until three a.m. When I awoke, I noticed Diana was missing. I got up and found her pulling an all-nighter on a metal bar stool by Kyle's side. We both stared at Kyle while he slept for almost forty-five minutes; I then went back to bed. I didn't have Diana's stamina. She is adept at missing sleep. I'm not. I was hit with a devastating amount of lassitude, especially after dealing with overwhelming emotion and a heavy dose of fear.

On the way back to the bedroom built for adult pygmies, I inadvertently ran into an old employee and friend, Angela. She had apparently been staying in the room next to ours. We hugged briefly and talked for a time. It seems her two-and-a-half-year-old daughter, her only child, had drowned in the bathtub while her husband took only a moment to answer the phone. She had been life-flighted to this hospital as paramedics tried to resuscitate her. Her daughter had arrived at the hospital in a coma. The physicians had tried everything to keep her alive, but her tiny body couldn't hold on. Angela was there picking up their things. I noticed how insensate and emotionless she was as she told me the story of her daughter. She was clearly still in shock from the intensity and sadness of her loss. Her eyes were red from crying, her face puffy.

I just nodded in response to her horribly sad drama. I had no idea what to say.

Even though she had just lost her own child, Angela asked about Kyle and his problems. She appeared genuinely concerned. I gave her a greatly reduced version of our day. She nodded and wished us the best. I felt inadequate to deal with her loss. After a last quick hug, she walked away.

Angela's situation hit me hard. Just when I thought we had it so bad with Kyle's tumor, someone showed up with a much heavier, much more depressing life story. They had lost a happy, completely healthy little girl within a few hours. In contrast, Kyle was still alive, with a vague promise of more time for him to run and play and grow. It was a somber reminder to be grateful for your blessings, even when times seem dark. Diana was next to me when I woke up. Her eyes were open and red. She needed to be held. I comforted her, holding her to me in that tiny bed, in that tiny room, through that long night.

19

Kyle's biopsy surgery was to be performed that morning. Dr. Bryson would remove as much of the tumor as possible and send the biopsy to an in-house pathologist, as well as to a more accurate out-of-state lab. It all sounded so orderly, yet overwhelming.

Diana asked a million of the right questions. Her Socratic persona overwhelmed the tremendous worry and fear that had formed a mask over her face. I stood by, helpless, as I nodded my head in vague agreement with everything that was said. I asked questions that had already been asked and answered. Diana's and my brains could not accept any of this as reality. To have a child in such a grim situation is a nightmare. It cannot be contained or solved. There are too many uncertainties.

The stress drained our lives and physical beings. Though we could have not slept enough the night before Kyle's surgery to hold on to an ounce of stamina, we stoically sat, worn out, waiting for more to unfold.

We waited a lifetime from when the orderlies took Kyle to surgery for the biopsy. I remembered later that day that I had tickets to the Harlem Globetrotters for that night. I had planned to take two of my sons, Kyle and Tim. It was nice to think about something so fun and normal. Things can turn upside down so quickly. I remembered my dad taking me to the Globetrotters when they played the Generals. It was a wonderful, cherished memory with my father. I thought about my two sons' faces, watching crazy basketball. Seeing the bucket of shredded paper, instead of water, being thrown out into the bleachers. Watching the basketball move around the players with grace and ingenuity. The sleight of hand. The silliness. Now, three tickets felt heavy in my back pants pocket, thick paper muddled in tragedy.

Our guts burned as we waited the hours that seemed like weeks.

Kyle came out of surgery and went into the intensive care unit. We followed his bed down the hallway. He was groggy and incoherent, but grinned at us with a soft, lopsided smile. His head was bandaged under his chin and around the top of his semi-shaved head. Drugs had taken his liveliness so he could peacefully rest. He glowed, sweet and innocent and unknowing.

We were told it would be at least an hour before we could see him. They formally dismissed us. Diana and I grabbed food from the cafeteria as he slept off the anesthesia. The food went down in lumps, scraping our throats and settling hard in our stomachs. We checked our cell phone clocks like mice on a treadmill. Each of us started conversations without taking them anywhere. We both spent most of our time inside our own painful thoughts.

After finishing our food, with forty-seven more minutes to wait, Diana asked me, "So what do you think of all this?"

Wow! A real question.

I exhaled, as if I were blowing up a huge balloon. "I'm not really sure how to react to everything. It's like it isn't real, and yet so overwhelming. Too much reality! We've been here barely a day, and so much has happened to our son—our healthy, intelligent teenager. I want to scream, but . . . I'm not sure what about. This is crazy!"

Diana looked worn down. I'm sure I had that same, dark look. She nodded. "Yeah, it is crazy. It is overwhelming! I want him to be all better. I want someone to tell me it's all a mistake, a bad dream. I just want to take him home and tuck him in bed. And . . . and I don't know . . . I don't know what to do."

Her eyes teared up. Mine followed suit. I wiped my eyes, feigning an itch on my nose.

We interlocked our hands on the table, staring at each other's lost faces. A buzz of conversations circled around us and plates, barely touched, waited in front of us. She would start to say something, hesitate, and then shake her head. I followed her lead and tried to talk again. Nothing came out. Everything was a blur——the world out of focus.

After thirty-five minutes, I said, "Let's go back up." It was one of those things I wanted to do, but at the same time, I didn't want to do. I wanted to know what was happening to our son, but I was afraid to find out. I kept inching forward in my seat.

We hurried to his room, and even with all the shuffle of people and medical machinery in the halls, we found solace in each other's presence. We headed together up the elevator, around the corner, and past the nurse's station at the entrance to the children's ICU. We clung to each other's hands in a white-knuckle grasp as both of us huddled inside ourselves. Like battle-weary soldiers, we waited in front of the desk for acknowledgment of our request—actually, more of a demand—to see Kyle. That is a hard thing to face, waiting for an unknown someone to approve of you seeing your own sick, helpless child, in a place of strangers and tubes and wires and monitors. We watched the nurse head in our direction and released each other's hands. The blood in our fingers started to recirculate.

"No. Not yet," said the nurse. I wondered if I bit through my lip when I heard this. Diana and I unanimously and instantly hated her for the relayed message. She was ugly, crude, and vicious. Reluctantly, we went to the waiting area to join all the other physically drained relatives in uncomfortable positions, nervously anticipating the double doors opening with news of their son, daughter, sister, or best friend.

We enjoyed the first breath of air when we were finally told we could see Kyle. We followed the nurse into the intensive care unit. Our hatred for her had diminished. The room was dimly lit; children in small beds were hooked to IV bags, their loving parents standing stoically by. Monitors displayed signs of fragile life. We had a moment of hesitation as we entered his space on the crowded ICU floor with it beeps, bandages, and the smell of hospital antiseptic and sickness. Kyle was sleeping. He looked peaceful and unharmed, other than a tube running from a thin arm to an IV and the bandage wrapped around his chin and head.

Diana held his hand on one side of the bed. I stood on the other side, rubbing his shoulder. Our hearts burst as Kyle opened his eyes forming drowsy slits and smiled in recognition. It was his own personal smile—the one we had watched for years had come back to him. And he knew us. Thank God! All forms of things are imagined when someone you love is going through brain surgery. How many neurons could have been lost? How much collateral damage was caused? Him recognizing us was such a relief.

He knew the question before we asked. In a loud whisper, he pronounced, "I'm okay." His head sunk into the pillow, and he fell back to sleep. We stood there by his side for a long time. Nothing much was said between Diana and me. We just watched him sleep, taking in the noises of other adolescent patients and their monitoring machines. It was a room of sliding curtains and tiny electronic lights. It was late at night, perhaps early hours of the dark morning. We didn't know or care.

Later that day, Kyle was finally alert enough to be told he had undergone brain surgery. He was asked all kinds of questions by the doctors, nurses, and us to check his memory. He was asked his name, his age, how many fingers the nurse held up, who the president was, where he was, and so forth. It was worrisome to watch as Kyle searched his mind for the appropriate words and thoughts with a look of concern on his own face, anxious to verify that he could still think, process information, and express himself.

We waited through all this with anticipated relief and concern as Kyle's normal self slowly came out.

Once the doctors and nurses were satisfied and left, Kyle carried on a game of sorts for a while, searching for various words to describe things, testing to see if he still knew the things that mattered to *him*. After a while, my wife handed him a stuffed dog that she told him his girlfriend had brought to the hospital for him. She absently asked him what it was. Kyle clearly and sweetly responded, "Meow?" then laughed at his own humor. Diana looked startled and worried before joining him in relieved laughter.

Having put his own concerns (and ours) to rest, Kyle then concluded, "Well, at least I still have my vocabulary."

Hospital time slogged slowly. Later that night, the ordeal sank in a little further, and Kyle became a bit agitated. He asked us, "How could they do surgery on me without my consent? I don't think they can do that, can they?"

Diana answered, "We gave consent. Don't you remember us talking to you about it?"

"No! I'm the patient. Why didn't they get *my* consent?" Kyle's eyes narrowed and his brow bunched up. He was truely upset. His thinking process had always been years ahead of his age. "They needed my consent."

We explained to him about parents' permission and their right to do what is needed for their children. We also explained how serious his situation had been with the seizures, and how the doctors had needed to act quickly. As we tried to reassure him, I could only imagine how upset he must be feeling. To wake up and find out your brain was operated on, without you even knowing it, must have been intense. We were patient and caring. Kyle finally understood and calmed down. He fell back to sleep.

By ten o'clock the following morning, they were ready to move Kyle to a regular room on the oncology floor. He was happy and talkative. He joked about the food. He ate it hurriedly, just like a teenager. He was full of life and seemed generally unaffected. He worried about schoolwork, the plans he had with his "girlfriend," and missing his normal routine. He wondered when he would be back at his junior high school. There was a Winter Jam concert coming up that he wanted to attend. Some of his relatives and friends from school visited him in the hospital, which made his day but wore him down, though he always kept his lopsided smile.

Diana stayed with Kyle twenty-four hours a day. I spent the long days with them. My late nights were spent at home, exchanging clothing for the next day and sleeping fitfully in a quiet house, alone. Diana slept on one of those crude chair beds in Kyle's room. Our son Jim was in the marines, stationed in North Carolina. Jeremy was in Montana, running wire for computer hookups through vacant stores at night. Tim was in school and staying with his mother, my ex-wife. Life was still moving forward.

On the third day of Kyle's hospital stay, Dr. Bryson motioned us out into the hall. We excused ourselves from Kyle and his visiting grandfather. It was morning. The snow reflected off the windowsill from outside as I closed the door to his room. The three of us huddled around the corner from the door, like covert operators. In unneeded whispers, Dr. Bryson explained the definitive answer on our son's biopsy results from the out-of-state lab. Kyle now had a tumor with a name: *Glioblastoma Multiforme.*

With a somber look, Dr. Bryson informed us of its aggressive and non-curable nature. Her demeanor and matter-of-fact clinical knowledge yanked away any strength we had left. Diana and I swirled in a fire of too much, too quick. We stood motionless and dumbstruck for several minutes after she finished talking. All of us stared at a spot, just below each other's eyes, not really breathing.

Diana slowly asked the question my brain wanted me to ask, but that my mouth refused to utter. I could not form any of the words. "How long does he have?" The question hung in the air for some time. No one moved. The air became molasses thick.

Dr. Bryson shuffled her feet and licked her top lip. "Well, as I said, GBM is extremely aggressive. You could have weeks with him, or months. If I had to estimate . . ." She paused, as we waited, then reluctantly continued, "I'd estimate three to nine months. I'm sorry I don't have better news. Some of the therapies will help. We removed as much as possible to relieve the pressure and slow the growth. We will do everything possible to give him as much time as we can."

Those time frames echoed in my mind. It was hard to breathe or swallow. I glanced through teary eyes as Diana wiped at her cheeks, her mouth trembling in fear.

The clock seemed to have stopped only on our lives. The rest of the world moved forward with sin, passion, war, floods, love, vacations, famine, and mail. Skiers traversed down slopes of snowy white. Bills were received and paid. Chairs were sat in. Indoor plants were watered. Television still blasted the absurd and the obscene. Our cataclysm was hardly noticed. Our life had been turned over and stomped on. Y2K had happened to us instead of to the computers.

After talking, we agreed with Dr. Bryson that it would be best not to tell Kyle everything, unless he asked outright. We would not lie to him, but we felt he didn't need to know everything.

It was one of the hardest things to do—to walk back into Kyle's room as though nothing had happened, as though no terrible information had been learned. I took two trips to the water fountain and three to the nurses' station for tissue paper for me and Diana before we walked in, following Dr. Bryson. She started a conversation with Kyle. Whether she meant to or not, it helped Diana and me through the weight of knowledge that had been dropped on our hopeful spirits. We stood barely erect, with forced grins and tired eyes.

The doctor told Kyle that he had a tumor in his head. She explained that most of it had been removed, and he would be taking medication to help with headaches and try to eliminate the rest of the tumor. She told him he went through surgery like a champ.

That was eight months before my heart attack.

20

Over the next week, our thirteen-year-old son began healing from neurosurgery. His horseshoe-shaped scar seemed to fade into fuzzy hair. Kyle recuperated well and was soon wandering around the hospital, making friends with the staff and other young patients.

The day of Kyle's release, he, his friend Kristel, and Diana went to the Winter Jam concert that he had worried about missing. It was a consortium of modern bands, playing one after the other.

The concert stoked him with excitement as he nodded to the music with surgical tape wrapped around his head. Toward the end, though, Kyle wore out; he fought exhaustion as long as he could, but the three of them left early. The next day, he couldn't stop talking about it. Family members thought we were crazy to let him go on the day of his hospital release, but we were determined to keep life normal.

After the concert, Kyle rested for a few days and then went back to school. Diana and I drove off to work. Nothing seemed to have changed, and yet everything had twisted in a new direction. He returned to his schedule of school, time with friends, a bittersweet growth of maturity, along with the new routine of frequent doctor's visits.

Kyle was a teenager who loved to toilet paper houses, build potato launchers, and tear electronics apart; they always worked perfectly when he put them back together, though several pieces and screws were still on his desk. He enjoyed hanging out with friends. Reading was one of his favorite pastimes. He was competent at homework. He had those stringy, loose arms and legs most early teens have. Kyle loved rock and country music, as different as they are.

He also had an intellectual humor that I always found striking and endearing. One time, I complained about a hamburger that had an inch of ground meat hanging over the edges of the bun. After that he always teased me about wanting very little meat on my burger. "Just ketchup, lettuce, and a fat bun, and you'll be fine," he heckled me. Even after full days of hospitals and blood tests, he always had his endearing smile.

Diana went into research mode, finding out everything available about Glioblastoma Multiforme, a new expletive at our house. She researched studies on medical websites. She made copious notes, blazing through yellow highlighters like a potato chip binge. She reported to me every night. Her office at work became a GBM center between her clients and court briefs.

Diana called clinical trial doctors around the United States. Each clinical trial was fastidiously rated based on duration, focus, phase, and results. Proximity had no bearing, except that it had to be in America. She discussed many of the options with Kyle's team of doctors—a neurosurgeon, an oncologist, and a radiologist. After a time, the team was considering three of the trials that might help Kyle.

An interesting chain of events happened at that point.

The local doctors had decreed that radiation followed by chemotherapy was the treatment protocol. We took Kyle to the radiology department to have a mask made. This was essentially a webbed cast to hold Kyle's head still while the machine bombarded his head in exact points, hopefully killing only cancerous cells. He took this lightly and found a bit of science fiction fun in all of it. He joked with his friends and his brother Tim about his horror movie mask. In fact, he even talked about wearing it for Halloween.

The mask made the cancer too real for me. It spoke of hair falling out and vomit and sickness. I had seen the television movies and read articles on cancer treatment. In my mind, radiation had no light side. It was simply an attempt to extend life by vile means. It was also a necessary evil to slow the growth of violent cells. It was what needed to be done. There wasn't much choice at the time.

Diana and I held hands. Diana endlessly twisted her hair. I tried to breathe through my constricted throat. We stared like lost souls into oblivion.

Once the mask was made, Kyle was to begin radiation treatments. Diana and I had adjusted to its inevitability and had figured out how to accommodate it.

When the time came, Diana took Kyle to the radiation department—the nuclear medicine department, as it is technically called. There was only one person ahead of Kyle. After they arrived and filled out the usual gluttonous pile of paperwork, Diana and Kyle were called in. Within a short time, Kyle was escorted into the room and began following the technician's instructions as they set him up for his first radiation session. After much preparation, he was left in the room alone, to be viewed through a window. A few clings and clangs—then silence. More buttons were pushed, and computer keys were clicked. Still nothing. The multi-million-dollar machine simply broke down. Kyle was released from his facial bondage. All appointments for that day were cancelled. He was rescheduled, leaving us a bit perplexed.

A Dr. Watson from the hospital called shortly after. He asked if we had thought any further about the three GBM trials. Dr. Watson had reviewed sixteen clinical trials Diana had asked him about, and he liked three of them. Two were the ones Diana had centered on. However, when Diana had asked the oncologist, she had been less than encouraging. Diana explained this to Dr. Watson, but he encouraged her to follow up. Diana then called the three centers involved and received a call back from one of them at Duke Medical Center in North Carolina. The trial was headed up by Dr. Sri, who had a much longer, completely unpronounceable name than that, so that's what he went by.

Diana spent an hour and a half on the phone with Dr. Sri the next morning. Thankfully, Kyle fit every requirement for participating in the clinical trial. The only item that nearly disqualified him was that he could not have had any radiation treatments. The machine breaking down turned out to be a miracle for us. God had favored us with access to the Duke University medical trials, which ultimately extended and improved Kyle's life considerably. It is amazing how sometimes things just fall into place as if someone helped. We believe HE did.

A week later, the three of us were flying to Raleigh-Durham, North Carolina. We carried the x-rays and a whole information package from Kyle's Utah doctors. I spent the night with Pepto-Bismol, gearing up for our visit to the Brain Tumor Center at Duke.

Dr. Sri's office was in an uninteresting building surrounded by thick patches of Carolina trees. He was friendly and knowledgeable, all handshakes and helpful concern. His dark complexion accentuated a youthful, alert face. Hand gestures followed each word he spoke. He put us at ease in a foreign setting, so many states away from ours. He explained that we would do testing that first day and a PET scan two days later. We would then begin the clinical trial with its therapy. The trial had thus far had wonderful results. Things felt right.

Diana filled out reams of paperwork then Kyle struggled through a half day of tests. We waited, reading bacteria-infested, six-month-old magazines—just like in the doctor's offices at home. Our outward appearance remained calm as our interior prayed about the hurdles Kyle would have to make it over.

The next day we walked with Kyle to the next section, more tests, and a new rack of old, overused magazines. The appearance of twelve hours of exam rooms and tests turned out to be four. We exited the clinic at one p.m. after a quick cafeteria lunch of brown and green food on a foam plate. I knew it would be another Pepto-Bismol night.

After a stop at the hotel, we headed to Camp Lejuene in Jacksonville, North Carolina, where Kyle's brother Jim was stationed at the time. Jim, a marine, was living off-base in a one-bedroom, one-black-puppy cottage, surrounded by a Carolina forest. There were many other cottages hidden slightly in the thick trees. Dirt roads wandered to each home. We caught up on family, episodes of interesting days, and life as a marine.

Free from hospitals the next morning, we jumped into our rental vehicle and headed east to the Atlantic Ocean. Kyle loved walking barefoot along the shoreline of sand, shells, and lost refuse. We wore sweaters and winter coats to keep the bitter ocean breeze from freezing us as we enjoyed the repetitive flow of rolling water. The sun was shining, but a cold ocean breeze kept the temperature down. I ran in and out of the water with a gasp and immediate pain, my red feet finding the sand just as cold as the water. I rubbed my throbbing feet back into organic flesh. Kyle frolicked in and out of the water's edge, simulating those scavenger birds with long legs, dancing with the tide on the beach. All this pulled us further away from dark thoughts of tumors and skirting the edge of death.

Two hundred yards from the icy beach, we warmed up and bought T-shirts and absurd scrap-drawer souvenirs from a colorful, high-ceilinged store called "Beach." The store featured a floor-to-roof wall of T-shirts, bags of shells, dried blow fish and starfish, and ridiculous things only a tourist could cherish. On vacation, even a medical trip, our traveling brains lose any wisdom, becoming frivolous and disjointed as we buy stuff we knew we would regret as soon as we unpacked at home.

We downed a late dinner on Topsail Island at a restaurant shaped like a lighthouse with a fake pier over a sea of asphalt. We had fish and chips in baskets lined with grease-absorbing, blue paper. Kyle became fascinated by the center attraction: a fish tank the size of a barge that displaced at least six tables. Swimming and crawling sea creatures had Kyle's head rotating and bobbing with glee. Fish as big as loaves of bread followed each other like baked bread on a conveyer belt. We headed toward the setting sun, back to our hotel in Raleigh, North Carolina, with indigestion from fat-filled, dough-crusted fish as we sailed swiftly along the freeway in an abused rental car.

Late the next morning, Kyle had a PET scan and more blood tests. We arrived early, so we walked around part of the campus. We found a delightful, tall building with spires. It was the Duke University Chapel. The chapel appeared to rise graciously from the earth, upward toward heaven. Inside, sculptured figures and stained-glass windows portrayed characters from the Old and New Testaments. We admired the quiet chapel for some time until we had to leave for our appointment. The chapel and closeness to God boosted us and livened our step as we headed to the clinic.

Reality returned. We received instructions for the five-day-dose of clinical trial medicine. Diana and I did the waiting thing as Kyle was given a psychological profile. We had prepared ourselves with paperbacks and snacks, all of which were ignored. Kyle was treated like a young prince, with everyone interested in him and his status. As we left the hospital clinic, he had sleepy eyes and a crooked smile.

Dr. Sri gave us instructions on administering the dreaded dose of clinical trial medicine. It was a chemotherapy drug called Temezolamide. It had been successful in treating breast cancer and had showed promise with GBM in a previous trial. Kyle would take the pills for five days, then wait a month, come back to the Brain Tumor Center at Duke University for another PET scan and blood tests, then return home to take the dose again. It was all very technical and medicinal, but it gave us a boost of hope.

By late afternoon, we were flying back to Salt Lake City. Exhaustion pivoted us on an edge between comatose and barely coherent. Our heavy eyes viewed the world through eyelashes. Light, relaxed breathing sung from our son's lips.

I tried to lift my book to read. It just sat there as I stared at the cover, willing it to lift enough so my sleepy eyes could pretend to read the blur in front of me. It wasn't worth the effort, and I wasn't sure what I would do if I opened it. I lost consciousness somewhere over the Midwest. Thoughts of tumors growing diminished into nothingness. Y2K, here we come.

21

I showered, shaved, dressed, had a breakfast of Raisin Bran cereal and V-8 juice, combed my hair, brushed breakfast and last night from my teeth, kissed Diana, held my car keys with an it's-about-time smile, then backed the car out of the driveway. It was the end of February 2001, and I was finally headed back to work after months of rehabilitation. Music flowed from the car speakers as I tapped the beat with fingers dancing on the steering wheel. Even bad music soothed me today. Cold air flowed past my left ear from an allowable one-inch opening of the window. I snickered. My mind wandered with anticipation from the duties of work to the traffic I was slicing through.

I held my chest as I hit the deep gutter surrounding the parking lot at work. I had also held it over every bump in the road, at each stoplight (whether red or not), and at each turn on the way to work. No way was my heart popping out through a severed rib cage held together with catgut suture and 22-gauge wire. Anxiety and elation glued me to the truck seat for a few minutes.

I had made it through a major heart attack, bypass surgery, recovery, and was now stepping back into some piece of normal activity. Gone were the mountain of pillows and the annoyance of a remote that, no matter how many times I pushed it, could lead me to nothing of interest. The door to getting on with life had opened.

I stepped out onto slush-covered asphalt. The air tasted wonderful this morning. My feet were instantly wet and my ankles cold, but it was nice to take the good with the bad out in the real world. My loafers filled with semi-solid water, and my breath hung before me with each exhale. I realized my coat was more decoration than warmth, but I whistled, happily slushing through the parking lot. On the purposeful, wet walk to the door, I consciously kept my hand off my chest. It wasn't easy.

My workplace smelled comforting to me. I looked around at ordinary things—furniture, carpet, and wall pictures—and enjoyed the feeling.

The top of my desk was orderly. Even the old-style, four-line phone looked polished. My normal stacks of scribbled-on yellow pads were missing. Clearly, the cleaning elves had been there. The built-in desk was old with an abandoned, used look to it. Deep years of scratches and polish looked back at me as if to ask, "Where have you been?" There were vacant in-and-out metal racks and an emptied pencil sharpener to one side. Everything seemed old and pristine.

Smiles and hellos echoed in my ears all throughout the day.

"It's good to see you."

"You're looking well."

"It's great to see someone here that knows what they're doing. We missed you."

I was approached with nice apprehension, as if I might shatter into small pieces at any minute. It made me uncomfortable. I even tried arguing over the phone with a supplier about things that didn't matter. He told me he would fix it right away and hoped I was feeling better. I wasn't. Physically, I was fine, but this kid-glove treatment was annoying and irritating and several other negatives with –ings on the end. Sure, I was dizzy and out of breath just from walking in from the parking lot and taking off my coat, but I felt fine. I probably had the pallor of a frozen Norbest turkey and the gait of a wounded sloth, but I was fine. Well, fine in a new way. Fine for a returning hospitalized person—slower, thinner, and readjusting.

My associates at work all told me how great I looked—the lying little bastards. I owned a mirror. I accepted the *new* me. I had evolved this far, so it wouldn't be too many sunsets before my color came back, my spine held upright, each step became brisk with intention. Let them tell me I look good and then silently wonder how soon my obit might appear. Things will change. The memory of my death walk will be forgotten. I will just be myself again—no pity, no grief, no sorrowful second glances.

I checked on back orders and reorganized a display of video cameras. I listened to the salespeople chat with customers. It was a slow month of the year. Christmas had come and gone while I was confined to bed. It was the retail lull after the year-end clearance sales and tax refund season when cash stopped flowing back into the store.

I had been in retail for years, which now makes me cringe. Retail is for people who don't have a life when everyone else does. You work moving inventory out the door every holiday when others are waterskiing, enjoying picnics under shady trees, and having wonderful conversations at family reunions. You work every weekend. Conversely, you get days off during the week when all your friends are hard at work. You get the privilege of talking to people who badger you into selling something for less than profit. You get yelled at by customers returning items as if you built the item in the back room.

February's end was a good time for a recovering manager to come back to work. I managed a retail furniture and appliance store when my cardiac arrest hit. I left for my first stay in a hospital just before Christmas. By the time I made it back to work, little had to be done. Sales were slow. It was the time of year when I made things up for the sales staff to do to avoid going crazy. The same thing hit every year. People had spent their money. They had lots of new gifts from Christmas and useless items from the clearance sales. Tax refunds were all spent. The store had walls of televisions flickering. Salespeople stood in endless boredom, talking about drivel and watching game shows as their brains kept breathing and circulation functioning.

My first day back, I worked at working. I had lunch by myself at a mundane place across the street, split-pea soup and half a turkey sandwich on pumpernickel. I had interesting conversations with a fair number of the employees. No memory of any of the conversations stuck. It was all inconsequential niceties. But after being at home for the extended recovery, it was great to talk to other human beings besides my wife. I love her deeply, and she is interesting, but wow, different voices after all those months bring on their own ecstasy.

I met with the corporate manager to discuss absolutely nothing at all. I reintroduced myself to the company computer. It was ancient, built sometime between the first color television and the Sony Walkman, about the time the game Pong was popular. The text came out yellow with blurred pulsing edges. It was unnerving to be selling state-of-the-art electronics and ringing the sale up on a computer with gear noises.

I drank a lot of water throughout the day and urinated most of the afternoon. Still, there were no abnormal colors. All in all, it was a good first day back to work.

The drive home involved tunnel vision and geriatric road speed. There seemed to be honking behind me, but my concentration was fixed solely on the path ahead. My peripheral vision was turned off, so I assume that the people in the cars passing me wildly were mid-finger waving as they went by. The journey was short in distance and protracted in time. The radio was low and between stations, though soothing somehow. With my hands firm on the wheel, my curled back leaning slightly forward, my face in total concentration, one foot on the brake, and the other on the gas, I stayed to the same lane of traffic all the way home. I signaled two hundred yards prior, then pulled my *rig* into the driveway. At least, it felt like a fourteen-wheeler to me. Even the steering wheel seemed larger and the gutters deeper.

I sat in the driver's seat, feeling the pressure slowly release as the drive home ended. I'm not sure why driving was such a task. I still had those unfounded worries related to my chest being held together with baling wire and suture. I had once watched an old Monty Python movie where a gigantic lady was fed pasta with a shovel in a restaurant until her chest and stomach exploded, leaving only dangling entrails and ribs. I was irrationally afraid of my own chest bursting upon the slightest impact from my car. I finally opened the door and got out. I arrived home without exploding.

The house was warm and comforting. The winter chill climbed up the stairs as the door closed. I giggled like a schoolgirl, for no reason other than the safety and warmth of my furnace-fed home. I was exhausted from the momentum of the day. Little actual work had been accomplished, but it wiped me out. The comfort of the couch surrounded me. I stared off into nowhere with thoughts of nothing meandering through my head—–it felt so good.

After an hour of my zombie-like state, Diana came home. It took me thirty or forty seconds to recognize her. I wasn't asleep, just distant.

She stared at me momentarily and then asked, "Where are you?"

I slowly responded. "Uhhhh, I guess somewhere far, far away. Mmmm, wow!" I shook my head to clear it a bit. "How was your day?"

"It was all catch-up and craziness. A two-hour deposition from hell. Clients calling and whining. Some days I hate my job." She blurted it all out quickly as though the whole thing was one word.

"So, it was a pretty average day?" I said, grinning, holding my chest with my right palm as I sat up.

"Pretty much! How about you? How was the first day back to work?"

"Kinda like I wasn't there. Very little got done. I had meaningless conversations with a lot of people. My time was spent trying to figure out how I should spend my time. I had brief periods with shortness of breath, anxiety about my chest popping open, and three pens didn't work. I wasn't sure what to tell any of my staff to do. Hell, I didn't know what to do, at least anything that mattered. But I am looking forward to tomorrow."

"Oh, you have big plans for work tomorrow?" The stress of her day was gradually melting off her previously tight face. A half smile was forming.

"Definitely. First thing, I'm going to throw those three pens away. Right into the wastebasket."

"That should fill your day until lunch."

"Only if I take a late lunch, smart ass."

She punched my arm.

Kyle watched from the doorway and grinned through steroid puffed cheeks. I knew he had been doing homework by the pen that dangled from his fingers. He made me forget about my pitiful problems just seeing him.

I turned back to Diana. "Speaking of lunch, how about dinner?"

"Sounds good. Do you want leftovers from last night, or should we do the ones from the night before?" she asked.

I leaned forward, bouncing up from the couch and giving her a hug. She went limp in my arms as if ready to give up for the day. I had risen too fast, so that ridiculous, lightheaded feeling sort of floated my eyes to the back of my skull. I gave up on the embrace and sat back down. After a few moments, I said weakly, "How about you choose?"

She picked the meal from the night before last. Microwaved to a sizzling mass, the lasagna and mixed veggies tasted wonderfully adequate. The three of us enjoyed a pleasant, silent dinner. We just nodded to each other once in a while and smiled. Kyle ate very little then headed off to bed.

I think we were all pretty beat that evening. It was a comforting relief for Diana and I to be on the same page.

Quickly, my routine at work required minimal intellect, several ounces of luck, and a pound of help from my staff. It folded into a neat package every evening and opened with meticulous care each morning. Before my heart attack, I used good inherent sense of what needed to be done, and I did it. But, after surgery messages were sent back and forth with way too much thought—neurons exploding, I spent more time analyzing work. I was becoming my wife, Miss Meticulous USA. These were uncharted waters for me.

But many things change when an illness strikes you down. Primary among those is one's outlook on life. Some people lean heavily on their God. Some close up shop and give up. Others begin daily exercises they haven't done since struggling in gym class as a teen with zits, insecurity, and lankiness. Some sign up for a zillion cable channels and cocoon themselves into a favorite ratty chair. Others commit to a life of overwhelming labor. The dietary bug infects some, so they watch every intake of calorie and gram of fat, both saturated and unsaturated. They use so little salt it becomes nonexistent, and dietary labels become their bible. Certain people just keep smoking and eating French fries, washed down from a well-stocked fridge of six packs. It affects all of us to some extent differently.

I took a middle-of-the-road approach to my new-found life extension. I stayed away from most fast food and dinner-on-a-stick places. I changed the cooking oil I use to olive or canola. I visited the gym for steady but mild cardiac muscle work, mostly treadmill. I wasn't looking to stain my t-shirt with triangles of perspiration, gain pecs that wiggle on command, or overdose on weights only to hurl afterwards. On the other side, I set limits on myself for the couch-potato time that enveloped me for long periods after surgery.

I shied away from my old bad habits, such as drive-through, deep-fried whatevers and farm-fattened red meat. I had a short glass of wine most every evening, while the empty bottle of Jose Cuervo stayed on the shelf as a bookend. I haven't smoked since I nailed my last pack to the wall with an angry hammer at twenty-one years of age, and that'll never change. As per doctor's orders, I slowed my gait when I walked. I used to move like the Road Runner on the Warner Brother's cartoons. Post-recuperation, my pace is more like that of Elmer Fudd.

Visits to the library and internet searches made me relatively knowledgeable about cardiac dos and don'ts. I also realize that scanning the internet for facts is not like deciphering the stone tablets Moses brought down from the mountain. One has to read five or more articles and find some congruency of truth.

Most living creatures adapt to changes. I don't think anything wakes us up more than illness, even if it's someone else's that we vicariously experience. It affects us, and we modify ourselves to survive, making it easier on each of us. If we don't, we're not around long enough to realize it matters. There is a reason there are not a lot of retired old gangbangers. They either change or they take a bullet from someone younger. The same holds true for smokers, alcoholics, and those of us that had some essential part repaired. It is crucial to extending our existence.

My work was a place of contentment and invigoration. The sense of accomplishment was greater and the rewards more profound than before my cardiac arrest. I would breathe in the air of simply doing and finishing. It felt wonderful. The beginning reminded me of a rough, pebbled road on bare feet. The walk was jerky, with no order. Each step was tangibly wrong and haphazard until, as if by the flip of a coin, I found myself making the right moves again.

It is very nice when you find your skill. It returns with vigor. It continues filling you with pride, success, and fulfillment. The neurons reconnect. The malady that put you in the hospital grows faint. Old work habits fall into place.

I began reorganizing things that were left behind. I made fastidious to-do lists, filling a whole yellow legal pad with scribbling, drawings, arrows, one, two . . . through whatever, with sub-sections A, B, C, D; subsections a, b, c, d, e, f; and references to previous thoughts. I wanted to skip lunch but gurgling stomach noises and faintness reminded me to eat and eat soon. I took my pad with red, blue, and black disposable pens to a Subway for a processed meat sandwich. Taking slurps and bites between filling more pages of my notebook, the stomach noises changed to tiny burps and the lightheadedness disappeared. My anxiety rose as I tried to write with fervor. I was back. This was the Jef that I knew. The workaholic was back, leaving behind the pillow-fluffing couch animal with saltine crumbs tumbling from ratty T-shirts to somewhere between cushions and a lost TV remote. This felt great. This was better.

22

We visited Duke University Hospital every thirty days for eight months between March and October. Kyle underwent tests and brain scans for a full day. We then headed to the beach to gather shells and enjoy the hypnotic surf, Jordan Lake to fish and picnic, the marine base to see Jim, or the sights throughout the Carolinas. It became a three- to four-day vacation and a one-day stop at the clinic. We made Kyle's therapy a fun adventure.

There were a couple of times we went boating on the coastal inlet in Jim's fishing boat. I called it "the floating wonder," because we always wondered if it was seaworthy and if the motor would start. Sunshine, sea water, and ocean use had eaten away at parts of the boat. It was like a comfortable old shirt, held together by thin strands of sun-bleached fabric, a shirt that always feels so good to wear. The motor gurgled, coughed, and sputtered before finding a rhythm and carrying us on our journey. I always looked to make sure paddles were in place. The steering wheel was so loose that as Jim turned the wheel, it wobbled about ninety degrees before catching. Then the boat floated into a gradual curve as a small wake followed. An inverted bucket was the captain's chair. One time, a metal brace fell off the rusted trailer. We had to wire it back on before loading the boat. A silent prayer helped us haul it the five miles to Jim's home. I watched as chunks of rusted metal seemed to fall off the trailer as Jim washed the saltwater off.

On one trip to Carolina we visited a butterfly museum where we watched those light, colorful creatures lifting and dipping with winged grace. It was a wonderful break from chemo and the clanging tone of the CAT scan and Kyle's somber face that smiled worriedly when he noticed someone was looking.

Another day we toured a historical ship at the dock off the Cape Fear River. It was the *U.S.S. North Carolina* Battleship

Memorial, a restored WWII battleship. Kyle, who always had an interest in how everything worked, pulled knobs and pushed buttons as he wandered like a pinball through that giant hunk of iron.

We walked various beaches and wandered as tourists in small beach towns. We tried to make the clinical trial visits seem to be an afterthought, with our focus on memorable fun times with our son.

The visits to North Carolina shrunk Kyle's tumor for a while, giving us a glimmer of hope. But his tumor was stubborn. By the eighth month, it came back with velocity. The Temezolomide quit working its wonders. There would be no more North Carolina visits. We were back to the standardized cancer treatments of battle and wait.

By October Kyle had begun radiation treatments. They kicked the cancer back for a while. He didn't lose much hair, just in the spots specifically targeted by the radiation. My wife shaved his hair on the sides and added inked paw prints walking around his ears. This was another attempt to make everything positive in his negative world. He loved those paw prints, and the young girls at his school, where the mascot was a bobcat, thought they were "So cool!"

At the end of November, I took Kyle to radiation. It was a few weeks after my heart attack. I was dizzy and sick. Kyle was happy and nonchalant about the whole tumor-radiation thing. He was worried about me, commenting about my hard breathing and fatigue. It was so like Kyle to think about others. As life took on a craziness, we both consoled each other without words. We struggled internally with our bodily fights and inner demons.

I knew my own circumstances, but I wondered how Kyle coped. He took things in stride as he physically and mentally changed. I worried about what pain lurked behind his crooked, pleasant smile.

23

After the heart attack, there was always a lingering shadow, whispering reminders to me about my silly impaired health. Climbing up and down a ladder brought on chest heaviness and short, panicked gulps for air. My natural, expedited stride of one foot in front of the other, which had moved me forward for almost fifty years, was a poison I drank every day. It was physically and mentally hard to walk more slowly, counteracting years of ingrained, quick, deliberate movement. Our own pace is imbedded so deep in gray matter and autonomic function that changing it is frustrating and almost impossible.

Hobbies I once loved became chores, interspersed regularly by stopping to catch my breath. I would have sensations and quiet memories of hiking up mountains, snow skiing down slopes of white puff, building things of wood and stone and concrete, scampering between the world of animals and cages with my children and grandchildren at the zoo, climbing trees with ease and attitude, and playing basketball with perseverance but little skill. Things had to be moderated. *Moderation* is an easy word to say but a most difficult thing to perform. I found both laughter and sadness in my new ineptness.

Weeks passed without any meaningful occurrence of heart or lung events. I wasn't 100 percent—but being stabilized at 75 percent felt wonderful. I was scheduled for an appointment with my cardiologist for blood work and several machine hookups. It's interesting to go into the doctor's office feeling okay. The visit seems almost wrong. What's the term? Is it called a wellness visit, or is it a healthy checkup? It's a hard thing to wrap my mind around when my history dictates doctor appointments only when something is broken and bleeding, something foreign is shooting out of an orifice, or a rash is so extreme and itchy there is no other solution.

My cardiologist's office was on the second floor of a building attached to the corner of the hospital where surgery had rerouted my blood's plumbing. It jutted out at a right angle, creating the illusion it had always been there. Perhaps it was the first building and the hospital came later.

A large, oval aquarium gave me pause in front of the reception desk. Two hourly paid receptionists waited on patients who were searching wallets and purses for insurance cards, the lifeblood of modern medicine. A short line of three of us waited nonchalantly for a spot at the desk. Americans are taught at an early age to stand in line and try to act patient, though the lip biting and swelling of impatience in the chest is closer to reality.

I waited for the third "next" to be uttered, and I watched the exotic fish darting about in the aquarium. I'm not sure about the biology of fish. If they have any intelligence at all, I am this unnatural environment must totally suck. One square meal a day of unappetizing colored flakes would make me want to run my head into the glass walls. Fish are supposed to eat sea plants and smaller fish, and they are supposed to be eaten by larger fish. It's hypnotizing and soothing to watch their graceful movements, but if there's any chance reincarnation actually happens and I'm destined to be a fish, I hope I'm too ugly and colorless to be put in a hospital aquarium with a plastic sunken ship and painted ceramic rocks.

"Next!"

I was prepared and handed my driver's license and insurance cards to the receptionist. She wasn't impressed. Her tone was an octave above condescending. Her questions were lazy and rote. Her expression was unctuous and seemed out of place given her pretty green eyes and light pink lipstick. As she looked at me, I received the fullness of her forced smile. She was young and in a mundane job but didn't realize it. After verifying with the computer, she was confident that I was who my cards said I was.

"Take a seat. The nurse will call you in a minute," came off her lips like dry sand blowing in a hot wind. If I was looking for someone to answer phones for me, her resume would be in a landfill by afternoon.

As I waited, I had also listened to the other young receptionist at the same horseshoe desk. She was pleasant and helpful as she patiently went over some papers with a seventy-something-year-old patient, adorned with a full head of gray hair. The receptionist's voice had a happy cadence to it. She seemed to take pleasure in her work and in helping the patients. It's amazing to me how two people can be trained in the same job yet be miles apart in performing it. I finished with my receptionist. I gave her a full, one-hundred-watt smile. She replied by trying to look around me to see if there were other patients to check in. Pity, she is just starting out; but with her attitude, she will probably be miserable most of her life. Hopefully, she just had a bad morning.

"Was there something else you needed?" she asked.

I realized I was staring. "No, I'm just dandy," I responded.

"Oh, then you're done, Sir," she said, nodding to the next person in line. I kept smiling and walked away. At least she called me *sir*.

I sat on an empty industrial couch. In front of me, outdated magazines with curled, torn corners looked up from a thin laminate, wood-grained table. This was the waiting room for five or so heart specialists and their staff. Chairs, couches, a window, and the obligatory pseudo-artistic paintings of European scenery looked back at me as I glanced around.

I was called in and weighed by a friendly, round-shouldered RN. She slid the weight bars over until she was satisfied, then jotted the number down on the clipboard. She slipped the clothespin-like gauge on my index finger to check my oxygen level. We stood patiently until it was 96 percent. I seemed to be standing and breathing with both lungs working. Good so far. She led me around a couple of corners and into the examination room. We had sociable conversation about benign subjects on the way. Her harmonious giggle helped me lose my growing anxiety.

My list of medications from my wallet was checked with their computer records to verify my chemical adjustments. My nurse was slightly doughy with genuine, happy cheeks and lovely eyes. We talked more while she went about her duties. I am always pleasantly surprised by people who genuinely care and enjoy their work. They lift you up. Most don't realize how much of a humanitarian they are. She was one of those.

My right arm was cuffed and tightened with the expansion of air, barely above the tolerable level. She straightened my arm out toward her and pressed the stethoscope end firmly down for a listen. She bit the tip of her tongue as she concentrated on hearing. "One-twenty-one over seventy," she told me. The nurse did the wrist thing for my pulse and punched her findings into the handheld computer. She disappeared.

Shortly, I heard loud wheels on industrial carpet from down the hall; they were getting nearer. The machine came through, banging into the door, followed by my nurse steering the cart haphazardly, as though one wheel wasn't turning. It was an EKG, one of many that have printed my record of up-and-down electrical heart notes. After plugging it in and pushing a button or two, she realized it was out of paper. My new favorite nurse excused herself, disappearing to wherever the paper is stored.

I had been here the day before for blood work. Something that is done with such ease and quickness hardly seems worth the drive.

My mind wandered back to a visit at my general physician's office, where I'm confident the phlebotomist came from the dark ages and practiced bloodletting. She drew my blood after several attempts to find a vein as if she was throwing darts at a target and mostly dotting the wall. Finally, a bullseye. A pad of cotton and a slap of tape covered my entrance wound with rough regard. My arm had tiny splashes of red around the tape. I wiped it off myself with a tissue from a box on the counter, put on my coat, and began walking out. I was relieved to have survived her industrial treatment.

After walking less than thirty feet, my arm felt wet. I yanked off my Italian leather coat. The coat lining and my arm were soaked in crimson—my blood, of which I had only ten pints. I could have filled a milk carton with what had run onto my coat. I grasped my arm and raced back to the blood mining witch, telling her I needed lots of cotton, rags, and leather cleaner. She and another girl from the back room raced to my side. The new girl held firm pressure on my wound while the bloodletter began cleaning the inside lining of my coat with rags. After several minutes, the bleeding ceased. I was wrapped with gauze and half a roll of tape pulled securely around my elbow. I sat for some time while the one who stabbed me with the needle continued to clean my coat. She did a good job of scrubbing. Perhaps she was only visiting from the laundry and happened to take a stab at my blood work. I was on high alert whenever I went back to that clinic. I'll never let her poke me again

Dr. Vandoven's nurse returned and hooked me up to the EKG with quick precision. She took a mound of tangled wires off the cart and separated them out with great dexterity. She attached each one with knowledgeable skill to the pads and machine and pressed the pads firmly to the usual designated areas of my chest, with one on my leg for good measure. In no time, she had the EKG spitting out a record of my heart's new electrical activity. I had been through this before. I relaxed as the machine printed out the secrets of my heart.

With a nod, she began ripping off the sticky pads, taking a few dermis cells and patches of chest hair with each. She apologized after each yank. I grimaced with each pull but said nothing aloud. Tight teeth ground into each other as she finished up. I watched as she left, playing battering ram with what was certainly an expensive piece of equipment. I heard it fading away down the hall.

A minute later, she leaned her head in with an angled smile, telling me, "Dr. Vandoven will be here in a minute," and left me to rampage through the room at will. I didn't. I sat and waited, looking around the room at medical pictures of the heart and lungs. They were interesting and boring at the same time. I had seen and studied each of them before.

I picked a magazine at random out of the metal holder on the counter. I thumbed through it, glancing at titles and pictures with little interest. Readjusting my butt to the seat, I began slapping my knee softly with the now rolled-up magazine. Boredom was settling in. As I have mentioned before, I don't wait well. I'm not sure many people do.

I tossed the rolled magazine at the counter. It perched almost on the counter. Dr. Vandoven came in as though entering a stage before a full audience. I was the only one there, so he shook my hand and smiled. "How have you been? You look good." He pushed the magazine to a more stable position.

"I feel good. I've been cut down a few notches with the heart and surgery being what they were; but, all in all, I'm doing okay."

He nodded his head and gazed at me as if I was incredibly profound. Both of us knew better. "Great! How about the meds? Any problems there?"

"There are too many," I answered.

"Well . . . at this time, we are not cutting any out. But, have you noticed any side effects from the prescriptions? Some are pretty strong pills, but we need to build up your cardiac function. Your heart suffered through a lot of trauma. It will take time."

"Trust me, I know. Every time I run up the stairs or set the treadmill above two, it lets me know that I have a defining limit. But, no, nothing crazy or way abnormal, like what happened with the Zocor. I am paralysis free."

"Good. Well, let's check you out."

We did the routine. I breathed in fully, swelling my chest, and then let the air out slowly as he listened to my back through the stethoscope that normally hung shawl-like around his shoulders. My chest scars were examined and kneaded. He glanced at my feet and ankles to check for any tumescence, made a few notes on his computer, and we were done.

"The lab results appear to be as expected," he said, lifting his brow with his fingers.

"I assume, 'as expected,' means good? You weren't expecting a bad outcome . . .as expected? I hope." I clamped my jaw down waiting for the reply.

"No, it looks great for all that you've gone through."

"Uh, doctor, that still sounds a little iffy."

"Nothing to be alarmed about. Your blood work is great. You are healing properly. Nothing is perfect; remember you just had bypass surgery and a heart attack prior to that." He stared at me, sitting on one of those four-wheeled exam chairs. He was sincere and helpful. His voice was quiet. His manner was unhurried.

I nodded my head.

"Any other questions?" He paused. When I shook my head, he finished, "Call the office if anything concerns you or if you have questions. I'll see you in two months."

After this checkup, I began a tradition of having breakfast in the downstairs cafeteria after my doctor visits. The food is well priced, chock full of cholesterol, quite mediocre, and is tossed sloppily on a plate. But it is institutional and comforting. I'm not sure why I enjoy the clinging and clanging of trays and sitting with so many blue cotton scrubs and people in various forms of discomfort, but I do. It may be the graduation from the cardio floor to the cafeteria, without saline being tube-fed into my veins from a metal coat rack on wheels. Whatever the case, eating there after morning exams and reflecting was a treat to me. I still do it to this day.

I went to Gold's Gym the next day for twenty-five minutes of low-level treadmill and ten minutes with light weights on a curl machine. Diana and I had signed up for a three-year contract during an outbreak of optimism. I knew the following day we may have overestimated our will and stamina, especially mine. My cardiologist had told us shortly after surgery that my heart, with only two-thirds of the muscle still functioning, would probably last about five or six years. I had a day or two of somber thought over those facts, but then my ego and my positivity kicked back in with elation. I was now determined to run treadmills for at least that long.

After a while of pretending to know a thing about exercise, we were offered a free trial with a personal coach. Diana and I had different goals. She wanted to lose weight and firm up. I wanted to survive by building up the struggling heart I had left. I needed to raise my ejection fraction. I wanted blood sloshing through my veins with the force of a fire hose. A sluggish, wimpy heart just wouldn't do.

Diana's exercise coach took her through measurements and structured equipment use. She learned the correct procedure for pulling cables, turning pulleys, and lifting increments of square, metal bars. She meticulously counted her intake with charts and graphs, penned quickly in a little notebook from her purse. She added and subtracted to find a calorie figure below her recommended amount. I kidded her that she was losing more weight from the energy she put into calculations in her notepad than she would lose from three or four days at the gym.

I, on the other hand, talked with the gym manager about my cardiac needs and limitations. He told me they had key people just for that type of task—physical trainers who understood heart conditions. He then introduced me to pubescent Brad after mumbling something to him about my existing heart ailment. Brad had the build and look of an Adonis—a bold-featured face; short, curly hair; a T-shirt that expanded with his biceps; two popped pimples with rub marks, one on his chin, one centered at the bridge of his nose; eyes of innocence and naivety; shorts four sizes too large resting carefully below the trim of blue underwear; and size fourteen athletic shoes with low-cut, white socks. He held himself in an unsure stance as he listened obediently to the manager. He was not far out of high school and, after talking to him a bit, I realized he wouldn't make it to college. I don't believe that all jocks have low IQs, but I'm fairly sure he barely burst through the single digits. It's a good thing respiration is autonomic, or I'm afraid he would forget to breathe. He did have youth and health on his side, though.

I was weighed and measured. They talked to me about body mass. The manager did something on a computer, soldiering back with a muscle-to-fat ratio. Mine was low, indicating little fat. I knew that from the mirror, but luckily the computer verified it. I'm thin, with muscles and veins that show. There are few soft spots. Those I have come and go weekly, depending on whether I ate pasta with heavy cream gravy or went for the walnut and pear chicken salad with a light touch of dressing. Next, they made a chart of my physical activities as questions were fired and Brad's pen filled the categories. I was marked from A to D, depending on a lot to a little, or by how many times per day. I assume I passed. No final grade was given.

The muscle ratio and physical SAT test out of the way, Brad proceeded to lead me through the rows of machines and sweaty, grunting patrons. He had me warm up by running on the treadmill. He set it way too high for cardio, but perfect to show off for some imaginary girlfriend I might have. As he walked away, I turned it down. I had read enough to know that heart patients need to start out slow and go for endurance. Pace the heart at a steady, brisk walk. This man-child knew nothing about heart conditions. The muscle-bound altar boy meant well, but he wasn't for me. Before leaving, Brad told me to run for ten minutes. I kept going for twenty. My understanding was that to build up the heart with cardio exercise at least twenty to thirty steady minutes were needed. Let's see—Brad was the expert?

My young trainer came back to get me after I had pushed the button for cool down. I stopped, and we walked over to the weight area. He had me do bench presses with way too much weight. I told him that much weight was ridiculous for a client who a few months earlier had his chest opened wide and then wired together. He seemed to comprehend, though he stood stunned for a few moments. He removed a great deal of the weight. I lifted it ten times. We rested. Then I lifted the weight bar twelve more times.

We moved to another area. Brad put me on a machine that simulated rowing against increments of weight. I was pleased. He moved the pin down to the second lowest weight. I noticed he was trainable. I began rowing to nowhere with even, long strides. He had me straighten my back. The seat moved as my arms pulled hard against the tide while the machine sat riveted to a cushioned floor. We tried a couple of other machines, with my trainer providing protective tips on how to use the machines. Then my time was up.

On the way out, the manager wanted to give me a high five. He raised his arm and, in football coach chatter, boomed, "Good workout!"

I let him keep his hand up in the air. With a subdued, deep-bass yell, I said, "Yea, great! That kid is a cardio master!" I flexed my arms in a curled, tight-fisted, mock "We're tough guys together" kind of manner as I walked out the door. I wasn't annoyed at the manager or at my so-called cardio-trainer, I just wished they really had a trainer who knew something about a heart patient's needs—or that they had been up front about *not* having a clue. I did enjoy the testosterone talk, though.

Humans in every form and nationality throughout the world want you to be more like them. The body builders understand you better if you want to be a body builder. The French people with their Eiffel Tower and Louvre museum want you to love art, be French, and eat as leisurely as they do. The wonderful people of Mexico learn Spanish and English from birth but feel far more comfortable conversing with others who speak Spanish. The educated are thought of as snobs, though they simply find peace in the language of knowledge, as opposed the vernacular of school dropouts. Rednecks are much more comfortable with other rednecks. People tend to flow with the river of least resistance.

We cannot be cookie cutters and molders of other people's experiences. It doesn't work. We each have the capacity for such great diversity. We acquire various needs from the environment and our genetics, making us the people we are. There is contentment in flowing with like participants, while diversity tends to let us wander out a bit and to grow, broadening our overall contentment.

I cannot be a body builder. First off, my restored pump cannot handle it. Second, I don't see the purpose. I find pleasure in my body being lean, quick, and strong. I have no aspirations to grow my body to proportions that require maintenance to keep it from turning to fat. However, I do enjoy running on the treadmill and pulling my arms against the strain of exercise machines to gain a healthier, better-sustained body. If I add muscle in the process, so much the better.

From that point on, I exercised by myself or with Diana on the treadmill next to me. I figured out what I needed as time passed. I knew my threshold. I added longer sessions and tougher trials as I worked my body up to it. If I became dizzy, which happened a lot, I slowed down or stopped and drank water. I was asked later why I hadn't signed up for one of the trainers. I answered, "When I decide to pump iron and head for the Mr. Universe title, I certainly will. But right now, I just want to be healthy and keep the clock working in my favor."

Those workouts made me feel so much better. I got lost in an unconcerned world of music and television monitors through ear buds. If I skipped a week or two, my attitude dipped along with my stamina. We have been told for decades to eat right and exercise. Who would have known it was actually good advice?

My natural pace and daily persistence were a form of exercise for forty-nine years. My nervous energy was given to me by genetics. It was taught to me by my mother, training at her side, keeping up with her gait that was barely under an all-out run. We raced through stores and backyard duties as though the hourglass was about to lose its flow of sand. She taught me the essence of grouping varied duties together in order to clean the house, make the lunches, weed the garden, clear the table, and dust the furniture, sparing little energy by never going over the same spot twice. If she was on her way to the kitchen from a bedroom, every bit of carpet lint and wayward sock was picked up on the way. There's a name for that kind of activity now—it's called "multi-tasking," and my mother was the queen of it before anyone knew what to call it. She had an economy of grace and speed, producing a beautiful blur of proficiency. She was my paradigm. Her example was the high-energy clay I was molded from.

My mom's movements had litheness to them, but it was not cardio exercise. It had grace with varied time frames. It was fast starts and spurts. Arms and legs went every which way in completing a project, with mini projects attached, all of it performed with seeming ease and great mounds of energy. There were never twenty to thirty minutes of concentrated heart rhythm on man-made machines. It was just my mom's nature to work quickly and steadily. I was the same.

I never learned about pacing the heart muscle to strengthen it. Gym class in school was all about flag football, full-contact basketball, and towel snapping in the shower. In health classes, we learned hygiene, and we could name bones like *femur* and muscles like *triceps*. Practical anatomy should be taught, though exercise of the mind and body is a wonderful asset.

It took my own heart attack for me to learn to be specific in my movements and careful in ordering at the restaurants. French fries and a malt taste incredible, but individual physiology dictates what it does to your arteries. Sitting by the pool soaking up the warm summer rays is wonderfully enjoyable, though swimming a few laps would be much better for the heart. We all tend to learn these things after the fact.

I continued to utilize the gym by myself, watching others to find new activities to do. My wife preferred the trainer. She liked someone to count reps and lead her to a healthier body. My workout was an experience of solitude and self-satisfying enjoyment. The separate ways worked for each of us.

24

At the end of February 2001, the inconsequential Y2K had come and gone, and I was feeling almost human. Kyle was done with radiation, and his blotchy skin was getting a much nicer tone to it. Our own funds were depleted from hospital machines and pharmaceuticals, and our inability to either focus on or arrive at work each day. We all desperately needed distractions.

Relatives came together financially and gave us an amazing gift of funds, making Kyle's life with cancer tolerable, yet meaningful and fun, for us and him. We worked on Kyle's own personal "bucket list" without letting him know that's what we were doing. We took a portion of the generous money we received and planned a trip with Kyle and his brother Tim to Cancun, Mexico.

The plane landed in Cancun, a city designed for tourists and the cash they brought. After customs, disoriented herding through corridors designed in the fifties, barreling through a barrage of tour sellers, and paying cab fare, we arrived at the palatial hotel. The cement construction was tinted beige, and palm trees stood like sentries lining roads and paths. We found a wonderfully overpriced Italian restaurant close to the hotel. The food was tasty, with perfect table settings on white tablecloths. It was quiet and opulent, until we arrived. Then the place filled with the excitement of two young boys, yielding unsettled smiles and having sword fights with well-polished forks. Eyes and gaping mouths harrumphed from the other diners. We were underdressed and over-hungry as we finished small portions, leaving with a slight growl still in our stomachs. At least the place settings were orderly and nice and the bill generous beyond belief. We dined on a bag of pretzels later.

That first night we chased waves back into the gulf. We drew ridiculous pictures in the wet sand and laughed with the freedom of vacation. Kyle and Tim took it all in with exuberance. Every minor thing was total fascination to them. They collected shells and chased long-legged birds. They dug in the sand. When that wonder lessened, they threw mud packets at each other before a mud fight erupted between all four of us.

The next day we explored Cancun, a city built simply to relieve tourists of bankcard-expendable limits. Our morning included too much breakfast; a weighted stroll with our new belly ballast; languorous beach time, reflecting sun off the brilliance of our natural white skin; thoughts about reading as the sun cooked our minds to a frail, unthinking mass; and downing colorful drinks that looked more like small fruit baskets. Thrown together, all of it robbed us of our ability to converse in complete sentences. Lassitude enveloped Diana and me. The boys poked in and out of the water, with little fatigue or slowing in their constant search for fun. After an unneeded lunch and a nap (needed by the parents), we headed into the city to eat again. Indulging in food and lying on the beach—what a life. It was good we only had a week, otherwise the weight gain and pure laziness would melt us into toad blobs on the floor. We would never stand on two legs again.

While I relaxed with a book, my wife worked on her list of restaurants from online searches and previous interrogation of friends. She had more recommendations than we could use in a century. She is always the fastidious pre-planner. I followed her with an air of what-fun-is-this exhale as we departed. She is usually irritatingly right, but I still prefer the haphazard, last-minute picks that drive her so crazy. We are such opposites in certain things; it's amazing we communicate and love each other so fully. At first, it was polite to adjust. Now, it is an adhesive that binds us together. For the most part, we know when to bend and when to be uncompromising. It works for us on date nights and vacations.

The restaurant was a place of fun and visuals. It was called "Carlos 'n Charlie's." The food was expensive and served by fun-loving college students on break, perhaps forever, from school. It was an outdoor place, something like eating on a gray dock next to a dark river. The lights flickered as if a generator were running out of petro. Tim and Kyle loved it as they watched the waiters bring out drinks stacked four and five high, balanced precariously on trays. They ate only a couple of bites of food, their necks twisting and turning. They were being sucked in by the excitement of the exotic surroundings. My wife's vacation planning had found a hit. Luckily, there was a flaw—closer to tip time, the waiter obnoxiously hovered and repeatedly filled our water glasses. He flirted with Diana and talked about "cool" movies with my sons. My wife found him adorable. He was tropical-climate unctuous enough for me to enjoy my bad hearing.

Diana whispered the amount of tip she thought he should receive. I shook my head. She gave me a look that could melt steel. I whispered a decent percent. She pointed up with her thumb and graced me with another of those looks. I shorted him by ten cents of her figure. She rolled her eyes. I know it was absurd, but that ten cents made sure neither of us won. As we walked away from the table, Diana tossed a dollar down on top of my tip money. Well, she won, and it cost us ninety cents more. I tried to give her a look. She smiled and sweetly asked with feigned concern, "Oh, do you have indigestion?"

There was band noise coming from the place next door. We decided to check it out. The boys were fascinated as they were pulled toward it by the sound of fun. It was a bar called "Senior Frogs." The bar was filled with eighteen- to twenty-year-old kids, drinking wildly, free from parental eyes. I have gone to similar places when I was in my late teens, thinking I was smarter than anyone over thirty, mixing drinks down my throat and into my stomach like a mad chemist, then spinning on a bed in pain for hours afterwards. It was carefree drinking, posturing, and hormone-dripping craziness in another country, where it always felt so much more mischievous. Kyle's and Tim's eyes were bulging and darting. Their faces were full of wonder and excitement. Never in their fifteen years had they seen so much erratic behavior in one place. And they were in a bar with eighteen-year-old people; how cool was that? The older girls, music, and the madness had them awestruck. I think they almost forgot their parents were there. We reminded them with finger twirls and watch-yourself looks.

There were young people dancing, high fives from Corona-littered tables shared by glassy-eyed students, drunk young girls sitting on top of tables, and the smell of alcohol and sweat and excitement bursting from happy, teasing co-eds. The beating music was decibels above the sound at most construction sites, and we tolerated the smell and shoe grab of wet-beer-sticky floors. The bar contained all the wonderment two underage boys could enjoy. We watched as teens took a tube slide from the rafters of the building to the inlet waters below in a screaming splash and hoot. The boys wanted to ride that waterslide but received an unmistakable head shake from Mom. I was so happy that Kyle stayed in good spirits with few headaches.

We found a picnic-type table. As we sat our elbows and butts down, the spilled beer glued them to the table and seats. Tables were probably washed after closing with wet, stained bar towels no more than every other Thursday. Diana got the boys and her some soft drinks and a Corona for me. As I sat, I noticed my hearing had improved—or maybe everything was just incredibly loud. I tried to shift positions, but I was loosely welded to the seat. I wondered what my shorts were going to look like from the back after picking up whatever it was below me. Diana and I talked about some positive lesson we could teach the two young boys but came up blank.

We people-watched for about a half hour, then I signaled Diana with a head nod toward the door. She agreed, and we peeled ourselves off the bench and proceeded out to the sidewalk. Our young teenagers kept their eyes alert as we pulled them out the door. They did not want to miss anything. They had a lot to tell their junior-high friends.

The night was well lit with a full moon and crowded bars. The traffic was unrelenting. Older teens were hanging out of windows calling out to friends they hadn't met. After we wandered aimlessly for a time, we found a cab and headed to the hotel.

I watched Kyle's exhausted, crooked smile in the streetlights as we headed back. He was having the time of his life—all grins and giggles. There is nothing better than watching your sick child be happy.

I was exhausted and my ears were buzzing as I dropped fully clothed onto a perfectly made bed. Sleep hit quickly with my tennis shoes on, a beer smell coming from the back pockets of my khaki shorts, and totally not caring what the boys were doing. Diana took on the duty of putting the three of us to bed. I was useless.

The next morning, we followed Diana's itinerary, taking a bus trip to a place she called Xel-Ha.

The idea of a bus trip made my head hurt. It sounded way too scheduled and touristy. There would be other people with itineraries and where-are-you-from questions, all dressed so casual yet eccentric. Being hauled on a planned-day trip reminded me of all those school field trips to hell where the teacher would discipline me for being a kid. Even if I was a bit of an ADHD child, being taken out of school to visit the outside world should mean freedom, not work release for prisoners. I spent way too many field trips sitting next to the teacher for me to enjoy any preplanned bus trip.

I have never believed in organized fun. It's like an oxymoron. The nature of fun is spontaneity and carefree meandering. How can you have fun if everything is preset and controlled? But that's my wife's way. I follow like a dutiful soldier because she usually has good instincts. Damnit.

Because of my wife's meticulous vacation schedule, we had three tours planned. I ground my teeth and smiled. She scheduled it so we visited the Isle De Mujeres by boat, traveled on a bus tour to the Mayan walled city of Tulum, and enjoyed the heat of another bus ride to Xel-Ha, which was a river-swimming tourist extravaganza. Xel-Ha was probably a peaceful Mayan fishing village way back when. The three of us watched as she daily went over her twenty-plus pages of restaurants and notations with yellow highlighters and some kind of numbering system; we called it the Diana Guide. Our stomachs growled as she asked what we thought about various restaurants and gave a synopsis on each. On certain restaurants we received more of a dissertation followed by a question-and-answer period. Kyle,

Tim, and I were careful to comment. She is a lawyer and would plead her case as though we had never had a meal before. She allowed me to have three gratuitous days of deciding our routine. That was a tooth-pulling exercise for her.

As I mentioned, I am a spur-of-the-moment person. I would decide at the last minute as the day progressed. Sometimes I would leave on an adventure without a clue as to where we were going. It drove Diana to a silent nervous frenzy. She wanted to gouge my eyes out—figuratively, of course—when I said the phrase, "Playing it by ear." I know what the expression means, though it doesn't make a lot of sense in today's context. It's like another expression I have used to describe my system of planning, "Flying by the seat of my pants," which sounds more like a non sequitur than any defining dictum. It has to do with intuition and previous experience. She believes it is hardly a way to plan a day. She is probably right, but I'll never admit it.

I chose the beach for the destination and the beach for the activity. I later picked restaurants based on their façade and any wonderful smells radiating out to the sidewalk. I also chose places to eat by the music they played, which had little to do with how well they prepared food, but it turned out fine. If the music was good and the beat strong, the food was fabulous, at least by my thinking.

"You should borrow my lists," Diana said.

"That takes away all the mystery," I responded. Her sober face and tight-lipped mouth told me to at least look.

To soothe her I glanced at it and said, "Thank you, that helps." Then I disregarded it. "We should be able to find something."

"We," she said sarcastically.

"Of course, 'we.' I'm sure the idea is pumping your whole body full of adrenaline with the very thought of it. I know how much you enjoy adventure."

"Yes, as long as it's planned out right," she said, fluttering her list in front of my face.

"That kind of dilutes the fun. Doesn't it?" I asked.

"No, eating unknown food from a restaurant with no reputation dilutes the fun. Dinner that ends in Pepto-Bismol and Alka Selzer is not fun," Diana said.

After a short walk, I said, "How about here?" I pointed to an older building standing by itself with the bright-colored stucco that Mexico is famous for. I watched Diana chew her upper lip.

She was regretting giving me three days. I regretted not having more. We actually had a good time with most of each other's picks. Our teasing passes the time, and she had her six days of rule; I had my three.

If it were up to me, vacations would be spent between eating at local restaurants picked at the last minute, relaxing in the sun, reading on a fine sand beach, and swimming the ocean currents. Sightseeing is neurotic behavior; tourist stops are mostly areas of extreme salesmanship and coercion. At those places, you buy things that end up in unlabeled boxes on high shelves in the garage. Really, how many singing stuffed frogs and glued shells in the shape of a pelican can you use? Obviously, with so many bursting boxes on your shelves, not many. I know people whose homes are so thoroughly infested with vacation knick-knacks that their great room becomes a Smithsonian of the absurd. Their walls define them and make them who they are.

I have a three-foot carved giraffe in my main room that I bought in Jamaica. As far as I know, there are no giraffes in Jamaica. I display the carved long-necked animal not to remind me of Jamaica, but because it is well crafted. It is one of the few things I have bought on a vacation with actual intent. Everything else is tossed or waiting for its day to be tossed from a box in the garage.

This vacation invigorated Kyle and us as we forgot about reality and health concerns for a brief time. Kyle and Tim were all smiles from the time we landed in Cancun to a week after we arrived home. It was better therapy than anything the hospitals threw at us.

25

Life proceeded as it always does, with an up here and a down there. The hills and valleys became commonplace and expected. Every few months I had checkups, blood drawn, and amusing conversations with my cardiologist. We talked about boating, hiking in the mountains, misperceptions of heart disease, news events, my cardiac progression, and the arrangement of large and small pills I swallowed each day. Sometimes he adjusted my medications. Sometimes not.

Things seemed to be good, but I was getting ready for a stent. My body just hadn't told me yet. Or I hadn't heard the murmurings from behind my ribs and cartilage. They were probably whispering to me in soft tones. I tend to be hard of hearing in many ways.

There were signals and signs my body gave off prior to my heart attack, but I passed them off as nothing. I experienced micro-sputtering and slips beneath my pectoral muscles that spoke of ongoing constriction and minute changes in blood flow. There were utterings, flinching, and spasms happening from time to time; I dismissed them as indigestion or normal getting-older quirks. I had brief moments when I lost my breath and gulped oxygen as a flush of scare flowed like an evil veil over my face and chest. I ignored them all, because they were subtle with little substance. It wasn't until the full cardiac tightening grabbed my back and shoulders that I perceived the impact. Even though my family doctor misdiagnosed the main event, I still had premonitions that something was wrong in Chest-Ville.

I had visited each of my parents when they were in the hospital for various heart problems and surgical procedures. I had completed enough college biology and genetics courses to realize the high probability of their passing on heart defects to me. I had been through many terrible weeks, lying in bed with leg cramps and a heart murmur as a young child with rheumatic fever. I should have known to expect heart issues.

Hindsight—what a ridiculous and late acknowledgment.

This time, I was heading toward one of the valleys of recovery—no energy. I was feeling terrible. Lightheadedness came easy. I knew something wasn't right. The dip worried me enough to call Dr. Edward's office to get checked. It was late; his office was closed. I thought about waiting it out, but my minor discomfort and shallow breathing caused anguish to wash over my wife's face. She hauled me to the emergency room. I went obediently on her leash of words.

I arrived at the same theater of craziness. I signed the papers the receptionist slipped under the glass after flicking specs of a Mounds candy bar from her fingers. She tossed the wrapper then photocopied my insurance cards and driver's license. There was no waiting, because I was a cardiac patient with tiny chest pains who sucked breaths in like a vacuum. An unsmiling nurse took my blood pressure and temperature. She seemed concerned and, at the same time, over-obligated. I was walked four feet to a wheelchair and driven thirty feet to the emergency room. The room was set up for utility—the gray unadorned utility of an empty closet. I looked around, then focused back on myself. I felt listless and blah.

A nurse with tightly curled hair maneuvered wires that lead to a monitor above my emergency room gurney. I was silently hooked up to an EKG where a printout purred. She slipped a finger clip over my right index finger to check my oxygen levels. It didn't work. I explained to her, as I do whenever they try this, that I have Raynaud's disease, which causes the fingers and toes to lose circulation in the cold—and it was cold. She nodded as though she understood and pulled it off, attaching the clip to my other finger. Then another. Then she tried my index finger on the other hand.

I finally held my hands out, palms up, in slight exasperation. "My fingers need to warm up. Reynaud's causes the blood to pull back from my hands and feet when it's cold. You cannot get a reading with all that vasoconstriction going on. Get me a warm blanket, and they'll work again. Then you can test my O2 levels. This room is Alaska."

The nurse clearly resented my irritated tone. But she raced off to get several warmed blankets. She returned, covering me in warmth. I rubbed my hands together to get circulation going. Sticking my finger out from the blanket, I watched as she snapped the finger cuff over the top. After only a few seconds, the blue screen monitor read 98 percent. After entering a note in the chart, the nurse hooked me up to an IV bag. She slipped out silently with a rear that shimmied down the hall. Illness tends to make me cranky and sarcastic. I want to be nice, but in a wounded state I have to work at it.

With my head floating, I felt nausea in my future.

My nurse was replaced by a nasal-voiced young man who drew blood with speed and expertise. He asked about the weather outside. Nice mundane topic. Diana talked to him. I ignored everything. He finished and scampered himself and the vials out the door.

An intern checked me over next. He made comments concerning my healing surgical scar, something about how well it was doing.

Yeah, great, I thought. *My lungs are holding up nicely*. I held my tongue, though, knowing my sarcasm rises as my health lowers. Instead, I gave him one of those let's-get-it-over-with yawns and sharp eyebrow raises.

The intern had begun listening to my chest and my back with professional intensity. He was not too far out of medical school, but he was thorough and concerned. He had no chin, just angled skin settling into folds from an inch below his bottom lip. He appeared more avian than human. His thin legs moved large, brown loafers in a sliding motion and held up his egg-shaped torso. He was a doctor still in the learning phase, so time was used up as he went through the procedural list in his head.

When you're ill, everyone always seems a little distorted, idiotic, and blundering. Things are just a touch off, settling hard in the annoyed category of life. It is difficult not to be a bit edgy when you're thinking with fear and scrutinizing odd pains.

Another doctor appeared in the doorway. He had a full chin hidden by long-shift stubble. The two doctors babbled back and forth in short medical terms I didn't care to comprehend. The unshaven doctor took a listen to my heart. I inhaled deep, long breaths for him, as instructed. He heard my lungs fill and expel.

The chinless doctor stood at ease at the end of the bed. He stared at my feet as though he had hidden homeopathic tendencies and was convinced massaging the balls of my feet would heal my heart. I watched him carefully. I pulled the warm blanket with my toes, breaking his foot trance. He looked me in the eyes, as if to say, "Why did you do that?" I looked over to the stubble doctor.

He told me they were going to call Dr. Vandoven and perhaps do an echocardiogram. I nodded my dizzy head as if I actually cared.

I lay uncomfortably as Diana held my hand, stroking what was left of my hair with her other hand. It became annoying, and I swatted at my head trying to extinguish the hovering bug. Her hand fell to her side.

"Is that bothering you?" she questioned, as if my hitting her hand was not message enough.

"Only a lot!" I answered.

"How are you feeling?" she asked, with pauses between each word and tenderness in her voice.

Somewhere between crappy and miserable, with a hint of anxiety to ride through it all, I thought. "I'm fine," I lied. I gave her a thumbs up that was feeble and listless.

She sucked in air, smiling at me. She was having a hard time holding that smile. "Okay!"

I was silent for a while, thoughts bouncing around in my head. I asked, "I understand the hospital wanting me here. You know, insurance payments and all. But why am I here again?"

"You don't feel well, remember," she said, without looking down at me.

"Yeah, that's the thing. I think I'm too sick to be here."

She leaned down close to my face. "Did you hear what you said? Isn't that statement filled with absurdity?"

"Well, I think I'm too sick to be here. I would be better off at home, letting it dissipate from my body."

"What? Do you think this is like the flu? It will go away in a day or two? This isn't a cold. You cannot just take Nyquil. This was your body, letting you know something is going on that shouldn't. You are a heart patient. You need to get this checked." She was emphatic.

"No, I'm way too sick to be here. I'm having an adjustment period. That's all. What I need is my own bed and a favorite book." I knew I'd be better off at home, but I also enjoy teasing my wife with statements that make little sense. Diana let out a stream of exasperated air.

She squeezed my hand a bit too hard and leaned too close into my personal space. "We are staying here until they figure out what is wrong with you. Just keep your head on the pillow!"

I sat up. "Easy on the hand, Miss Steroids; my IV is going to pop out and my bones turn to dust."

She released my hand and backed her face away from mine a couple of feet. "Sorry!"

"Jef!" Her face was becoming flushed as she went on. "You are definitely staying here until the tests are back. Now, lie back down." Her voice had raised an octave or two. She had formed fists, and I could tell she wanted to pummel me. She commanded, "Down, now!"

I hesitated and then lay back onto the pillow with a sigh. "Down, now, huh? Boy, you get easily riled. But, tell me, wasn't that a lot more fun than lying here listening to the monitor? For a minute there, I thought you were going to make me feel a lot worse than I already did."

Diana flapped her hands. "You were just playing me? You think that's funny? You find that sadistic humor interesting? You are a shit!"

"Honey, I'm very sick. Remember? Let's wait for the doctor." I paused. "Could you fluff my pillow?"

She repeated her earlier assessment. "You are a shit!"

Diana softly punched me in the shoulder. A finger pointed into my ribs. "If I fluff your pillow, it will be over your mouth and face."

"Shhhhh! The doctors are coming back."

She turned. There was nothing. Her face scrunched up, and she was clearly intending to use her meager vocabulary of expletives on me. Diana's mouth opened and contempt contorted her previous beautiful face. She paused, blew air out, and then just smiled at me, shaking her head.

After a few seconds, she leaned down and kissed me on the forehead. "Now be quiet, before I forget I love you."

I opened my mouth to say something smart-alecky. I thought better of it, and let out a soft, "Okay."

The clock stalled.

Finally, there was a knock on the shut door.

The unshaven doctor walked back in. He looked at us carefully. "Did I miss something?"

I answered. "Oh . . . no! Did you get any results from the blood test?"

"Most of the tests are back, and I talked to Dr. Vandoven," he answered in broken words, as though pausing for emphasis. "He will be here soon. He wants to personally verify your status."

"That doesn't sound like you are releasing me yet."

"No, Dr. Vandoven knows the patterns of your heart better than anyone."

The unshaven doctor spoke as if reading a script for the first time. I'm not sure if he thought I was slow to understand, or if he slowed his speech when he was unsure of what to say and how to say it. He also raised his voice a tone as though speaking to a child. It was infuriating. Again, I was sick. I felt like speaking to him in stressed, accentuated words, explaining the meaning of each verb and noun as I went along.

Diana broke the short silence. "So, what have you found at this point?"

"At this time, it may be nothing. Or, it might be a small blockage in one of the arteries feeding the heart. We will know more when Dr. Vandoven arrives."

I awoke an hour and a half later to Diana and Dr. Vandoven nudging me from both sides. My name was being repeated incessantly. In a groggy state, I said, "I was in a deep, deep sleep." I shook my head and stretched my arms a bit. "Wow! Where have I been?"

Someone else was in the room—a faded figure off to the side. I tried to reorient my eyes. Sleep was reluctant to leave me alone.

Dr. Vandoven said, "We are going to give you an echocardiogram and see what that tells us. This gentleman is here to take you for the test." He pointed to a man in blue scrubs who looked like he was about twenty. A gurney awaited me outside the room.

Diana followed as I was pushed through halls. This was a déjà vu. Ceiling tiles and fluorescents whizzed by. I was exhausted from hospital life—they could have done any test or procedure they wanted—a puppet without strings.

The frigid, sterile room woke me up. My gown was pulled down, exposing my chest sprinkled with light hair. Ample amounts of cold goo were applied to my chest and then spread around with the scanning end of the machine. Everyone looked intently at the screen. My heart contracted and pumped, again and again, beating with life on the screen. I always feel amazingly alive when I see my heart working on that small screen. The channel is always the same. When it changes, you're dead.

My cardiologist walked over and patted my shoulder. "We may have to do an angioplasty. We need to have an angiogram done so that we can verify what is happening. It appears that one of the arteries is 70 percent blocked and another is about 50 percent blocked. The nurse is checking on scheduling for the procedure. Hopefully we can do it today or first thing in the morning."

I ended up going home and coming back the next morning for more fiddling with my heart and veins. I was neither excited nor repulsed by the procedure. Sometimes numb and disinterested is the best you can do.

The next morning the hospital appeared congested as usual with people wandering the halls or waiting for elevators. All had urgency on their faces. I was signed in and directed to the now-famous waiting area. A miracle occurred, and the wait was short.

A nurse had me put on the open-back gown, always a crowd pleaser. Diana bagged my street clothes. *Hopefully I will wear them again,* I thought. On the ride to the room, I the only conversations I had were in my mind.

The queasiness of sterility and antiseptic fogged the room. A drone of cool air pumped into a well-lit but somewhat hollow space provided background noise. The nurse stopped and pulled the lever to lock the wheels on the chair as I stood up to walk to the table. Hospital-sock-covered feet echoed softly off aseptic white walls in concert with the sliding motion of my feet. The nurse led me as I shuffled with the posture of a noodle. For once in my life, my ego had disintegrated. I became an obedient, worn-out dog on a leash. Too much hospital does that to a person.

My teeth chattered. Goose bumps lined my skin in rows as arm hair stood at attention, and I glanced to see my breath as I forced it out, looking over my nose. I understand the part about bacteria having a hard time growing and thriving in a cold, refrigerated environment, but hospitals seem to have a way of taking it too far. It was for my own good, so I shivered and accepted it. The nurse brought a couple of white, thin blankets and cocooned me in. I looked at her as one of the great saints. As the warmth seeped in and the shaking ceased, I relaxed, laid my head on the pillow that smelled of bleach, and forgot where I was for a while.

I was surrounded by silver-necked lights, stainless steel machines, and gas hookup points with color-coded bands hung like silver moss off swamp trees. The nurses scurried, attending to me with blood pressure checks, shaving my groin, and attaching hospital paraphernalia to my limp body. Dr. Vandoven talked to me briefly, and I was injected with a relaxing drug. He had his friendly smile on. I cannot recall a thing we talked about. Hopefully it was inconsequential and I revealed no life secrets.

The monitor showed x-ray views of the dye going in, and the shape of my heart was brought into view, with capillaries and veins reflecting their presence. The metal wire holding my chest together stood out, appearing as three motionless, butterfly shapes within my chest. Shortly, I felt a slight sting as the probe was inserted into the vein in my groin and up toward the offending, misplaced matter. It's interesting that the best way to your heart is through your groin—which brings up all sorts of questions about love. Finally, the drugs became more powerful than my attention span.

I awoke to being slid over onto a gurney by a gaggle of shadows. My optics seemed shielded as I tried to gaze through weighted eyelashes. My eyes opened and closed in movements like those of a broken garage door opener. The chain was slipping. My arms seemed to be held down with invisible ropes. There was no dreaming, just the electric hymn of fluorescents.

Dr. Vandoven worked his board-certified magic, using modern science and technical skill. A stent or two were inserted and erected. It was a blur to me; I was in and out of the deep-freeze room in no time.

Back home I recuperated quickly. With slight rejuvenation, I had the weekend to stretch and laugh. It was as if nothing had happened. I was back at work on Monday. Of course, I had to live with the pubic haircut. A nurse always shaves one-half of your pubic area for the angiogram's insertion point—enough said.

The stint procedure went well. *Procedure* sounds so routine and common, like vacuuming the carpet once a week or doing the dishes. To me, opening a vital vein to my heart seems like a much bigger deal than that. It was life and death. I've vacuumed a rug that's a bit dusty with specs of lint, but vacuuming has never been critical. It is just a procedure I do every so often. I'm not going to die from dust allergies, though I may cough from time to time. A stent procedure hits me with the word *critical* all over it. I'm not quite sure where the dividing line is between procedure and surgery. But inserting a stent certainly seems a bit more invasive than a simple procedure.

I would have four more angioplasties after the first. I would receive several more stents to open vessels and improve blood circulation. One would be a routine "procedure." The other would be an anomaly, and my heart would struggle through it from the moment the dye was injected until several days later after recuperation hell.

Some people gain vitality after an angioplasty. It provides immediate relief and a rise in their energy level. For me, it helped my heart get a little better each time, extending my mortality. It was physical and psychological healing without instantaneous results. My body seemed to heal slowly and carefully, almost unnoticeably.

The heart is a crazy machine, all muscular tubes and bellowing, contracting chambers, synchronized and musical. With poetic rhythm, the heart pumps life fluid, containing carriers and infection fighters, a system of waste disposal, and self-sealing coagulants throughout every intricate part of the body. There are only five quarts of blood in the human body, reaching miles of passageways to feed and clean every cell so they can divide and multiply, continuously refreshing the body with new cells. What a miracle machine we have in each of our chests. I wish my car worked as well. Of course, it hasn't been in the shop as frequently as I have—at least, not recently.

26

I routinely visited Dr. Vandoven every three months for blood tests and an exam. Sometimes my prescription dosage would change; other times, the pills themselves changed. My heart was beginning to stabilize (whatever that means), and I was learning the things I could and couldn't do. I struggled to accept those things. Shortness of breath was a drag. Galloping up the stairs and skipping every other one in a race to the top left me lightheaded, my lungs burning with each breath. Ladders were out of the question, as were long workdays. After complaining to Dr. Vandoven, he told me to "simply slow down." He said, "Do the same amount, but at a slower pace, and be mindful of it." He also said something about not being twenty anymore and having this thing called heart disease. Illness is such a bummer.

Sometimes we are so caught up in being who we were, we forget to be who we *are*. I needed my doctor to tell me that. I must be leaving my common sense packed in one of those boxes on the high shelves in the garage. I went home feeling somewhat stupid. And rightly so.

Illness is such a bummer. Just when you think you're better, you must adjust to a weaker presentation of yourself. It creates other problems, both psychological and physical. The body adjusts, but the mind has a hard time accepting the inevitable—heart disease, kidney disease, osteoporosis, lung cancer, breast cancer, and so on. No one likes to be less than they were, but even the process of aging does that to us. Acceptance seems to be the key. I can't do it. Can you?

I worked on learning to walk slower and take my time getting things done. I had to mentally remind myself to pace my movements. Like the scorpion in that old story, it was against my nature. It was truly hard. I found when I didn't follow the gait of a DMV employee, I had to sit down, catch my breath, and wait for the angina to subside. That gave me reminders, but it was a hard sell anyway. It was like telling a smoker to quit. Of course, a smoker knows smoking is bad for them, but they light up first thing in the morning anyway.

Diana and I took turns taking Kyle to his various doctors' appointments. He had a full basket of them. Kyle saw an oncologist, a radiologist, a family practitioner, and a neurologist. All were concerned, friendly physicians who related well to a young teen and his chest-pounding, air-gulping parents. It turned into a routine habit. But the reality was never routine.

Our days were filled with either taking Kyle to his doctor appointments or me to mine. It was a strange way of life. We tried to balance things that should have made us all depressed, but we took things in stride and moved on to the next appointment.

I had turned fifty, and my regular physician, Dr. Martini, suggested I get a colonoscopy. I was in his office for a sinus headache. Yes, even people with major diseases get colds and flu like everyone else. My forehead pressure evaporated only when I was sleeping, and it kept me from doing that. Yet I tried to sleep continuously to subdue the aching frontal lobe. I asked if the colonoscopy would "clear my sinuses."

Dr. Martini laughed, a thing of rarity with him, responding, "No, they are completely independent, unless there's research I've missed."

"Well, I read on the internet where massaging a certain part of the foot can dissolve gall stones and that smelling certain herbs can help people lose belly fat."

My doctor rubbed his chin then held out the palms of his hands. "Jef, you realize the internet is wonderful, but it's also famous for outright lies and absurdities."

"I am easily amused. With the newspapers fading out, I'm sure the internet will be the funny pages of the future. Sometimes it's hard to differentiate the knowledgeable articles from the gibberish. But I enjoy both."

"Information is only as good as where it comes from," he retorted. "Now, fill this prescription and if it doesn't help within ten days, come in and see me again." With that, he turned and exited smoothly and quickly. I was dismissed. He was busy.

Enough with the banter; just take your meds and be gone. So, I exited with a script and a card for a gastroenterologist.

A month later the door to the gastroenterologist appeared larger than normal. The doorknob grabbed a bit, as if it was stuck and slightly higher than it was supposed to be. As I entered, a counter with hair behind it greeted me. The receptionist was short. I stood back and talked to a well-maintained hairdo and eyes with long, overworked eyelashes. A clipboard was slid out with papers for me to read and sign. I knew the routine. I pulled out insurance cards before being asked.

The doctor stopped by for a brief reassurance visit. It was welcome, though seemingly memorized. He had a pleasant nature, speaking with smiling lips.

Diana stared at me. I stared back. What do you say to each other before a colonoscopy? Our minds were blank. Blowing out gulps of air was our only communication, for once.

A nurse came in and gave me a shot of something to "make me relaxed," as she put it. I knew I would shortly be visiting Never-Never Land. She started to wheel me out to the procedure room. Another nurse, this one outside the door, grabbed the foot end of my gurney. I looked up at her. She smiled a Julia Roberts smile—grand, pretty, wide, and inviting. As the drug took over, her teeth appeared to grow a wingspan. *My, but what large teeth you have, grandma*, I thought. Her smile expanded exponentially from Julia's. It was inviting and grotesque at the same time. I lay, tense, holding firm to the bed rails for fear an inhale would Moby Dick me inside that cavernous place of tongue and jaw and giant, perfect, white teeth.

Her nametag proclaimed G-something RN—maybe Gouda, like the cheese, though I wasn't sure if it was her first or last name. If I were to pick a lineage, it would be Armenian. She was the nurse for my colonoscopy, efficient with getting my vitals without saying more than a few words. When she did speak, sentences came out in soft breaths. I expected more power from that mouth. I could barely hear her.

The other nurse had departed without a sound.

Ms. G-something's lips breathed a hushed, "Dr. Randall will be in shortly." A quick swivel of hips and bounce of hair, then she was gone.

I was alone in another antiseptic-smelling room, on another top-padded, white bed with a pull-out footrest on what I assumed to be the front. I tasted the bleach from the white sheet I was laying on. I looked at wonderful landscape pictures, a décor like I would have seen in an upper-class hotel, without the candy mint on the bed.

I had been given a sedative. I accepted the lightheadedness and the release of thought brought on by wandering, body-numbing chemicals slithering through my bloodstream. Even heart patients need a colonoscopy when they reach the magic fifty. There are television ads about it and billboards proclaiming the devastation of colon cancer from celebrities who regretfully waited. Magazines explain how simple it is, accompanied by physicians whose pictures look quite concerned. I think gastroenterologists and proctologists must have gigantic advertising budgets.

It's like Christmas. In the early days of America, Christmas was a simple, Christian holiday, marked by a nice dinner and the family getting together. Gifts were apples and nuts. Macy's changed all that by reinventing Saint Nicholas into Santa Claus and advertising all the gifts that everyone needed from their store for Christmas. Soon all the stores were advertising Santa, reindeer, and Christmas trees with a bounty of gifts underneath. And look what it is now. Christmas lights and gifts are in the stores by September, and there is an advertising push for yet another four months of buying frenzy. Black Friday has slowly crept backward to a flimsy point somewhere right after the first leaf falls from a tree. Thanksgiving is now just another busy shopping day. All of it stems from stores playing on needs we didn't even know we had. We never knew we wanted a colonoscopy either, until advertising advanced it to a need like the wrapped gifts under the decorated pine tree.

However, I do believe a colonoscopy and other preventive medicine is a positive thing. Anything that detects and prevents cancer cannot be a bad thing. It is amazing, though, that something we barely talked about and then only in whispers a few years ago is so mainstream now. Of course, things change. It has only been about ten or so years that we have been inundated by feminine hygiene TV ads. I never knew there were so many smiling women exercising happily during their period. I know my wife has never appeared to be having that much fun during their monthly cycle.

For a full day prior to the colonoscopy you can have only clear liquids, and you drink a bitter, foul-tasting solution. Your day is spent primarily in the bathroom, flushing your "system" and the toilet continuously. You feel completely drained (no pun intended) and mentally bewildered, deliberately drinking something to give yourself diarrhea—and the prize is a stinging sensation every time your bowels sing. The preparation is hell. The "procedure" is easy. Humiliation is just a cloud that passes. Fortunately, you rest unknowingly while the physician and his nurse are staring at your butt.

Later, the doctor, with glasses balanced on the tip of his nose, relives the experience with four-by-six color photos of the inside of your colon. Like a sightseeing guide, he explains the coloring and any imperfections or concerns. As fascinating as they are, you will never be as excited as he. Pale tunnels where waste flows will never be the snapshot of the month in *Photography* magazine.

The thumbs-up for no cancer or major problems was the only thing I cared about.

I was sent home with my memorable internal pictures. I was not sure when I would have time to frame and hang them, or where. I considered with distorted humor the pages of our old family album. "Here's our son when he was three, and my colon at fifty." The scattered room I call my study seems appropriate, but, no. They slid quickly into a drawer no one would open. Why I saved them, I'll never know.

I may have a semi-functioning heart, but at least my colon is perfect, and I have the pictures to prove it.

I find it interesting; I can count on one hand my visits to a doctor in my pre-heart-attack years. Now that I have endured the bypass surgery and associated conditions, I seem to see doctors once a week, and they know me by first name without looking at the chart. I used to get inconvenient illnesses, such as the flu or a cold, and think nothing of them. Now, every tiny gurgle in my stomach sends me heading to a clinic for blood tests and x-rays, as if each innocuous slip from the norm is terminal. Such is the situation with having a major illness.

I have become one of those dread-filled people, perceiving nothing as something and something as something else. My leg hurts; pain is emanating from joints that have lost their liquidity. Instead of understanding that something is age related or perhaps a slight arthritic condition, I view it as heart related. I get a tickle in my throat and then a cough, and I wonder if it's a heart problem or just a simple cold. I labor too hard on a bathroom repair project, and instead of acknowledging a stiff back, I become obsessed by thoughts of my original heart-induced back pains. I become illogical until I mentally slap my face, saying "get real." This behavior is probably common for patients with life-altering conditions. We fantasize over the trivial. It is a lot more interesting and damaging.

I should have paid attention to some of those oblique moments. There is that hindsight thing again. Though I am by no means brilliant, I have enough working neurons to consider what my body may have been telling me. There are signs. There are insignificant changes in our bodies so subtle, yet so loud, that we miss them.

For me, there was a realization sometime after my cardiac arrest that slightly conscious burps and shootings from my heart had happened, and I had given them less than a second's notice. I was a bit preoccupied with life when the fluttering motions of my heart were telling me the plumbing was becoming clogged. I had no idea my cardiac veins were screaming for help as angina pectoris was evolving. Angina is like being strangled and gasping for air. It is the protest of strangled, blood-carrying veins, trying to deliver cardiac-sustaining oxygen and nutrients to the ever-working pump.

A whole list of pre-heart-attack symptoms had shown their insignificant and mean, tiny heads for a few years prior to the "Big One." I list these not specifically as telling signs of cardiac problems but more as something that will help you know your body and pay attention to those small knee-jerk symptoms that are easy to disregard or blow up. Sometimes the body just reacts to new foods or environmental or psychological changes. Other times it informs us of things to come.

1.   Shortly before my cardiac arrest, I became fatigued easily. The exhaustion felt different—I needed to sit down, then lie down. I could fall into deep sleep during the day at the hint of any tiredness. This was a whole new world from my normal ADHD personality and energy level. I was used to going—going and doing and doing more. Naps were for other people—the weak, the sickly, and the intoxicated. The change made no sense, though I took it in stride, accepting it as the minor biological change of age. Now I realize my body was talking to me. Yelling at me would be more appropriate, but my simple brain failed to process the message. There should be a mandatory college course on listening to your body. I had no idea it even talked. I was too busy with life to even listen. Ironic.

2.   I learned about another cardiac event after the fact. *Ventricular tachycardia* is a rapid-fire pulse or heart rate. It gives you the sensation of tiny pains and flushing. Your heart speeds up, as though you were running and stopped to catch your breath. I remember specific instances of it. Driving in the car, waiting in line at the DMV, trying to pick out spicy mustard at the store. These all came back to me after the fact. It was a little late, but the memory is there.

When it happened, it scared me and made me wonder in silent exclamation, *What the hell!* I found an explanation for each one. It was the sausage pizza, or the garlic cream sauce, or too much pot roast. I would just pick a food from the previous meal, and that would be the scapegoat. Sometimes indigestion is just indigestion, except when it isn't.

3.   I had bouts of dizziness, loss of breath, and weakness. For me, the weakness part came mostly after the heart attack. Shortness of breath and lightheadedness were common just months prior to my attack. They were subtle but made me stop whatever I was doing and wait until they passed. They were brief, unlike the ones I received during and after my heart attack.

They were an annoyance, quick to happen, then vanishing with the same speed. I assumed my loss of breath and dizzy feelings were preludes to an illness coming on. I was thinking more of a cold, for which I needed to get plenty of liquids and rest, than a major heart condition with bypass surgery and a diet of no more fast food.

4.   There was one symptom of my looming heart disease that I thought nothing about. I had been in and out of hospitals with this staring me in the face, but I missed it. It's heredity. Both of my parents had heart problems. My dad died on the operating table with massive heart trouble when he was about the same age as I was, but genetics didn't even cross my mind. My mother had two heart valve surgeries. I inherited my parents' personalities and facial features, though my memory failed me when it came to all those nail-biting times of waiting for their surgeries to end. They had given me a little bad with all the good. All those weeks visiting them in cardiac wards never took on significance for me until I was in the ER answering questions about other members of my family and their medical history. It was a large, flashing warning sign, and I missed it.

5.   I also had times of insomnia and anxiety. But with someone as high-strung as I, it could have been my norm or a symptom. Hard to tell.

6.   I also had moments of short-term nausea. I attributed those to anything other than a serious condition. The queasiness would hit and be gone a minute or two later. It was merely another irritant, something I never related to my heart. Maybe it wasn't. It was so brief; if it hadn't happened numerous times, it would never have been memorable. I should have paid attention to it anyway.

7.   Medical researchers say muddled thinking is another pre-heart-attack symptom. I never had muddled thinking. If I did, I wouldn't admit it. It is too distasteful to believe I was ever a muddled thinker. If I was, how would I know? I'm not asking anyone about it. My wife would probably joke with me, saying, "You have always been a muddled thinker." I would find no humor in that, so I haven't asked.

It wasn't until after I began healing—when I started googling heart, heart attack, coronary bypass, vein, and a bounty of other prompts—that I realized the symptoms I had ignored as annoying irritants and inconvenient bodily burps were warning signs.

There are probably many other symptoms I either didn't have or didn't notice, percolating in the background like coffee before the full boil. Most of us never notice the symptoms until after the water already bubbles over the top. Hindsight is too late. We all feel invincible, until we realize we're not.

27

I was noticing physical improvement each week. There is no better feeling than that. I treated my cardiologist appointments as a necessary survival technique. Work was getting used to me, and I was getting used to its rigors. The steering wheel had not been a thing of demons for quite some time. I was still holding my chest in the palm of my hand, but with less frequency. My damaged body was feeling normal to me.

I had not yet begun the process of missing my old health. My ability to skip steps as I hurried up the stairs in days past had changed. I used each step and thought about my stride all the time, except when I forgot. At those times, my heart reminded me in very certain terms. I relished my advancement since those beginning days after leaving the hospital, when I struggled to walk the thirty feet to the end of my driveway.

I had been back for some time to a level of stability, creeping close to my former self. I was able to focus more fully on Kyle and his struggles with chemotherapy, steroid pills, hospital visits, teenage awkwardness, and school. I had always been there for him, even on my worst days, but bad health consumes energy and disposition. It was wonderful to gain back some life and the ability to be a father instead of a patient. Kyle's situation took me on paths away from my own longitude and latitude. I felt now I could focus more on his needs than my own.

Kyle now gave me his half smile through puffy cheeks as I dropped him off at his junior high school. He was filled with an inner happiness at doing standard things, like going to school.

Kyle had become something of a hero at school. All the students had watched him adjust to the transformations the tumor forced on his body. They viewed him as a fighter. He was incredibly smart, articulate, friendly to everyone, able to converse with the teachers at an adult level, helpful to anyone who was troubled or discontent, honest, and brave beyond reason.

When the drugs and tumor took their toll and his legs started tiring easily, Kyle received a wheelchair to circulate the halls at school. The prettiest and most popular of the girls fought over which one would push him to the next class. Sometimes he had two or three fussing over him as they walked him to his locker and his classes. According to several of his male friends at school, he was the envy of most boys. They were there for him also, as friends are. The times I drove him to school, a group formed around him with smiles and laughter, moving toward the entrance as a teenage amoeba, with Kyle as the nucleus. His face and previously skinny body were swollen from the steroids, but that never deterred his large circle of friends.

He was lucky to be well-liked and cared for at an age where someone different can be shunned and abused. Kyle had a persona that invited the good part of others to shine in full force. He had a gift of being pleasant and likeable without eliciting pity over his situation. He grinned and joked, even when his skull was throbbing with pain.

There was a time when Diana and I talked to one of Kyle's teachers. He was a history teacher who was not currently teaching Kyle in a class. Kyle had found out this history teacher's wife had cancer and was having a bad go of it. The teacher told us that Kyle always asked about his wife and sympathized with him. He said Kyle consoled in a way that always made him stand a bit taller after their conversations. "I never thought a student could teach me so much about caring," he said.

This was a time of drug trials, vicious therapy with caustic chemicals, and watching sadly as Kyle's face puffed so much that he looked like a different young man. There was a period of hospital travels across the country and to the other side of the city and tasteless cafeteria lunches at oncology clinics and children's hospitals. It was months and months of spending hours in uncomfortable chairs, waiting to visit medical doctors we knew well enough to address by their first names, though we didn't. We had seen these doctors so much that we recognized their shirts and blouses from times past. To be honest, that was a little unsettling. Obviously, there were too many visits.

Through all this, Kyle always kept his genuine smile and humorous wit. He knew his life would be cut short, but he refused to let that get him down. Each day he faced life as an adventure of familiar friends and interesting acquaintances. He exemplified sunshine and ebullience, insight and spirit dancing. I tried to be his mentor, but he became mine. I watched him smile when I knew he was in pain. I listened to his laugh when his eyes told me his stomach ached and writhed. For all the internal bodily turmoil he must have been going through, there were no outward indications of any problem in his personality or disposition.

I, on the other hand, took my heart ailment to gentle moaning and an indicative shudder or two. I found that point of volume on my moaning dial just audible enough to elicit sympathy, without really expressing the threshold I was feeling inside. I advertised my pain. I let my wife know each time I felt my heart misfire and even some when I wasn't sure it had. She endured my list of intricate ailments from the time she arrived home from work. I startled her every moment when I sucked in a breath and grabbed my chest. I was animate and vocal. I wanted to be a Kyle, and I tried, but it wasn't in my nature.

At first, she was consoling. After a while, she finished my achy-breaky heart sentences for me. She would occasionally even walk away with indifference, saying, "Yeah, it sounds terrible. I'm still listening." I would stop talking when she left the room. She never returned for the rest of the story.

I wasn't always looking for sympathy when I talked to my wife about my tiny pains. Mostly, I was just talking out loud to help me understand what was going on. She is a smart woman, and I wanted her comments and opinions. I also knew she would research my ailments and give me a full report. My research was more of a scan; I got approximations. She got details. While I could have done without some of those details, I appreciated her feedback.

After a while, I began talking to others about my cardiac experience. I used the same basic stories. Everyone knew someone with something like mine, so they shared those stories. Most of them didn't make me feel any better, because most ended with someone dying. I'm not sure why people think a good story has to be terminal, though those stories do have more impact when everything turns out okay.

I finally learned to back down from the day's events of sharp pains and gurgling spasms. Mostly, I came to terms with the episodes. They no longer made me wonder. They were just me. It was like inhaling or walking. They were just things that happened. Mystery solved.

28

Kyle's fifteenth birthday was coming up. We wanted this to be the best birthday ever—especially since we weren't sure how many more he would celebrate.

Kyle's puffy face gleamed with excitement. He passed out a boxload of invitations to friends at school. He and Diana planned the food and cake. Our house began to be cleaned as if the president of the United States was visiting for dinner. The house was taken apart and put back together. Furniture was moved from one place to another and back again. Our place smelled of ammonia and wood polish. The fridge was loaded, cake baked, candles purchased, and hands slapped if they touched anything that might be part of the festivities.

Kyle's body was swollen from steroids. He had lost some of his equilibrium and had to use a wheelchair to get around at school. He endured horrible headaches. Yet despite all these, he smiled and joked around as if life was filled with chocolate chip cookies and sunshine. He sat in a chair happily waiting for his birthday party to begin while Diana and I skittered around the house taking care of last-minute details.

The doorbell rang, and a stream of teens flowed into our organized and spotless home that Friday evening. Trays of cookies, brownies, and fudge were laid out on the kitchen table. Soda cans bobbed their silver heads through the ice in tubs. Goblets filled with M&Ms were laid strategically on each coffee table and end table throughout various rooms. Within a half hour, sixty-plus kids fused with sugar and excitable adolescence wandered aimlessly through our home in chaotic array. Kyle's eyes lit up like released balloons. More teens came. The entire school student body seemed to have landed at our home. The yard, front and back, filled with groups as the house burst at the seams. A traffic jam happened as parents dropped off more teenagers shrieking with excitement. Neighbors locked their doors and pulled their window blinds tight. Fear glistened through the neighborhood.

There were four adults—me, Diana, her mom, and her best friend. Needless to say, we were overwhelmed and understaffed. We kept refilling trays, hiding breakables in our bedroom, wiping up spills, and considered calling in the national guard.

My eyes widened, my chest tightened, and my heart pounded at my throat. Several kids scooped fingers of icing from the uncut birthday cake. I smiled as if everything was normal. Nickleback and Nelly rattled the walls with their lyrics. Three fifteen-year-olds with recently developed breasts were hopping M&Ms from the left to the right and howling with laughter at their accomplishment. Snakes of hand-holding friends wound their way from one room to another in some kind of rite of passage dance.

I eased my way through the young crowd to BBQ hamburgers and hot dogs, knowing full well we didn't have enough supplies to feed this whole group. The grill kept me outside where buns and meat disappeared as fast as I could cook. I spotted Kyle several times as several girls ushered him around, arms daisy-chained together. His amazing smile could have lit up New York for a month. This craziness was so worth it.

29

Kyle's lopsided grin became more exaggerated, but never left his face. He radiated warmth and friendship. His lanky body gained soft, fleshy bulk. He was having difficulties with balance and strength, but seldom complained. He would grimace and then say, "It's nothing, just a little headache." Diana's and my heart sank as we watched each little change.

Life went on.

In early June 2001, Kyle's laugh was contagious as we drove up the mountain road with the boat trailing behind us. Kyle and two of his older brothers, Jeremy and Tim, exchanged humorous stories about previous boating adventures. They laughed. Most of the stories featured me as the focus of the joke. They seemed to recall every silly or stupid thing I had ever done.

Tim started it with, "Remember when Dad almost tore the boat apart when it wouldn't start at Yuba Reservoir? We all jumped ship and hung out on the beach. He was pulling out tools and yelling at the motor. He was stomping and splashing from the front of the boat to the back."

"Yeah," inserted Kyle, "and mumbling about what we kids had done now!"

"And then," Tim said, "after half an hour, Dad realized he left the boat in gear and that's why it wouldn't start."

Kyle added, "His face was beet red."

"I was sunburned; my mind was scorched from the rays," I retorted. "And you guys exaggerate things."

"Sunburned, huh?" Jeremy stepped in. "We were only on the boat an hour or so. It wasn't even noon."

"Oh, but the best was at Strawberry Reservoir with that first boat," Kyle exclaimed. "The one Mom and I got him for Father's Day."

I said, "The sixteen-foot, wooden v-hull you guys paid a hundred dollars for, that cost me over a thousand for the motor and endless time sanding and refinishing?"

"You loved working on that boat," Kyle said. "You would hardly come in for dinner."

"Yeah . . . I know," I responded.

"But, the real thing with that boat," inserted Kyle, "was its maiden voyage."

I said, "I think we're all tired of that story."

"Yeah, I bet you are," said Tim. "We put it on the water. It started right up. It took off from the dock."

"And the boat would only turn right," Kyle exclaimed.

Tim added, "We had to drive it around in circles, always to the right. I didn't think we would ever get back to shore. I was getting dizzy."

Everyone except me was giggling, snorting, and cracking up. I looked over at the three monkeys, each doing different impressions of driving in circles. They really found this dad-bashing funny.

"First of all, you didn't get dizzy," I responded. "Second, the boat also went straight ahead. It just wouldn't turn left. And third, the stupid steering linkage was attached wrong."

"Let's see now, who hooked up the steering linkage?" asked Jeremy, a sarcastic smile on his face. The boys all did high fives with each other.

Kyle stated, "We had invited my uncle and his family from Omaha to go boating. They had fun watching your boat go around and around. Tell me that was not the funniest thing ever."

They all laughed again.

"Yeah, it was kind of like riding a dog that was chasing its tail," I said. "But the next weekend we went out, and it worked perfectly, thanks to my ingenuity." I patted myself on the back over my shoulder. There was momentary quiet in the truck.

"That and a lot of four-letter words," Kyle said.

They continued father bashing as I drove. I turned up the radio, though I was smiling inside. The radio didn't seem to help.

We were boating today at a mountain lake called East Canyon reservoir an hour's drive from Salt Lake City. It was a hard pull up the narrow, winding canyon pass. Cliffs and boulders dropped almost vertically down on one side of the road. Green vegetation squeezed its way through cracks in the rock. On the other side, steep mountains, thick with trees leaning into the sun, encroached on the worn asphalt. Runoff streams crossed the road at various points through corrugated metal piping. You could feel the velocity of vehicles going the opposite direction as they slid past, just a few short feet away.

The canyon is beautiful, especially in the early morning as sunlight passes through the leaves and branches. That morning the sun strobed to the music and drowned out the laughter and boating stories my three boys were enjoying.

East Canyon is a high mountain lake. The water is clear and frigid, even in the hottest part of summer. A hook and worm bring out Kokanee salmon and Rainbow trout. The fish broke the still waters as we backed down the ramp. It was peaceful and calm with a soft, hot sun mirroring clumps of trees around the lake. We had the lake to ourselves except for two tent campers and an older motorhome. It was decorated with dents, off-color patches, and lines of silver duct tape holding it together; it seemed better suited to a junk yard or being pulled by a tow truck.

Jim was the only brother missing. He was still at Camp Lejuene, off the Carolina coast, protecting the country, learning military expletives, hiking through thick forests, and drinking beer as an art form. Kyle talked about him and the fishing trip they went on together down the Intercoastal waterway. They didn't catch anything. Their lines tangled on underwater reeds while the sun baked their arms and faces. The aged boat trailer fell apart from seawater corrosion when they got home, but they had a great time together.

We hadn't come to fish. The poles were left idle at home. We came to boat and swim and enjoy a day together. Tim was the first one off the bow with a scream and a splash. Jeremy followed. I stuck my arm into the frigid water, deciding that today's swim was a young man's sport. I don't swim unless the water temperature is in the eighties, which never happens in this lake.

Kyle was content to watch his brothers swim. He smiled, leaning back on a Dolly Parton life jacket. I could tell he didn't feel well. He was usually the first in the water. Kyle never complained, but his silence shouted tons. He had a quiet stiffness to him and an expression of forced happiness on his face. It hurt inside to watch him suffer with that smile on his face—such a brave child. The other brothers pretended the bitter cold water was fine, despite the goose bumps and uncontrollable shivering.

After an hour on the boat, we headed to shore for some lunch. Tim and Jeremy barbequed hamburgers on a grill, unwrapped store-bought potato salad, and cut open the Doritos bag on a picnic table. We ate Viking style—no plates, no napkins. The boys began to eat. Kyle was back and forth to the bathroom. I think his headaches were getting worse. His eyes squinted in pain.

Kyle was bad enough that he finally allowed me to go to the cinderblock and cement outhouse with him. He told me his head felt like it was exploding, and the pain was making him sick to his stomach. The joking from outside with his brothers had ceased. The mountain birds chatter still stilled. A cloud shadowed us. Feeling Kyle's pain, his brothers became subdued and quiet as they turned the burgers on the grill. I held his shoulders between vomiting and diarrhea. Kyle was taking it in stride; I was a mess. After approximately forty-five minutes, he felt more at ease. He was still slightly nauseous, but his face had relaxed. I had him drink water, which was about the only thing he could hold down at the time. His brothers, for him, pretended nothing was wrong, though I watched the worry spill from their eyes.

We cut the day short, loaded the boat, and headed back down the winding mountain terrain. I had to get Kyle back home. Hopefully, we would boat another day. He acted as though it was no big deal, but I knew he did not get sick that often. The cerebral cancer did a lot of things, but the overwhelming headache that had hit him was actually unusual. I was worried. He thanked me for taking him. I hid tears behind dark sunglasses.

It was a much quieter ride back down the canyon. Kyle curled up beside me and closed his eyes. My throat tightened.

At home, Kyle rested more. He drank half a glass of Sprite and had a few bites of a croissant roll. He fell asleep on the couch shortly after his meager lunch. I calmed as I listened to his consistent breathing and watched his relaxed face.

He felt much better after twelve hours of sleep.

That next weekend, Kyle went to his biological father's home for a family reunion in Mount Pleasant, Utah. Kyle was excited to visit with his grandparents and extended family he hadn't seen in a while. Diana gathered up his pills, which was a task in itself. She wrote down specific instructions for his father to follow on pills, fluid intake, food, and care. Kyle packed his suitcase with clothes, games, and books. We met Kyle's father in a Wal-Mart parking lot; after hugs and kisses from us, he was driven to Mount Pleasant. We went back to Salt Lake.

A week passed. Then on Monday morning, the day Kyle was supposed to come back home, we received a call from his biological father. Kyle had been having terrible headaches all through the night. He had been fine through most of the family reunion and had even started a food fight with his aunts. But Sunday night he had apparently become so sick that he didn't know where he was; he tripped over his little half-brother, stumbled around the house in the middle of the night, and ran into furniture.

Diana and I had just left the house in two vehicles to return an Expedition we had decided not to buy. Diana organized a plan to meet Kyle at Primary Children's Hospital in Salt Lake City, where an oncologist, Dr. Belcastro, was alerted. It would take his birth father and family an hour and a half at high speed to reach Salt Lake, two hours if they followed the speed limit. We assumed they would arrive in the first time slot. We dropped off the Expedition and headed for the hospital.

We waited in the lobby. Our eyes scanned kids in various stages of fear and malady stroll in and out, their parents with dark circles around their eyes. Kyle arrived after a twenty-minute wait. He came in a wheelchair, his head bowed toward an orange plastic salad bowl held in his lap. He glanced up with a distressed, tired face. He tried to form a smile when he saw us; it turned out to be more of a pained look.

It was June 25, 2001, seven months after my heart attack and almost seventeen months after Kyle was first raced to Primary Children's Hospital with seizures.

We went straight up to Dr. Brugger's office and clinic in oncology. She was waiting for him and responded immediately. Kyle was taken to an examination room and injected with medication for his swelling tumor and scale-ten headache. They promptly had blood work drawn. His face was puffy from the steroids, but his lopsided smile returned as Diana and I held his hands. Everything happened within a few minutes of his arrival. We waited. We had hopes and tears.

Dr. Belcastro came out and signaled for us to follow her into her office. Kyle's biological father and his wife followed, and the four of us waited awkwardly together in anticipation. The room went quiet. Dr. Belcastro told us, "We're near the end. We'll get the pain under control, and Kyle will probably be able to go home tomorrow, but you'll need to get home health care set up for pain management. We're within a week or two of the end."

My mouth was dry. My throat felt constricted. I closed my eyes tightly to hold back tears. There was no response or question to what we had just heard. We stood and intermittently stared at each other and the floor.

We made our way back to Kyle's exam room and waited by his side for the pain meds to take effect. Kyle kept falling in and out of sleep. Sometime later, he woke to say his head and stomach still hurt. Diana rushed to get the nurses so they could give him more medicine.

An hour later, Dr. Belcastro evaluated him again. She told us in the hall that things were moving much faster than expected. It appeared today might actually be his last day. We had sensed this in our hearts, but the words were so frightening and real to hear.

Diana and I had known this time would come, but there had been no way to prepare for it. I put my arm around Diana, and she snuggled to my chest with sporadic sobs.

Kyle's oncologist broke the silence, letting us know he would be transferred to a special room in the hospital, and we should call anyone we felt should be there. She assured us they would make certain he would have no more pain, and she went on to tell us how things would proceed. Dr. Belcastro had done this before, but I could tell it was never an easy task.

Somewhere along the line, I called Kyle's brothers and other family to let them know what was going on with Kyle. Tim showed up shortly after. Jeremy and Jim were living out of state.

Within a short time, Kyle was moved up to a regular hospital room. His half-brothers and half-sisters arrived soon after. His swollen face looked peaceful as wet eyes filled the room.

I rubbed his shoulder and, unconsciously, my healed chest incision at the same time. Dr. Belcastro knew of my heart problems. She swiftly crossed the room to make sure I wasn't having a heart attack. I told her that when I get a slight case of angina, I rub my chest. It helps psychologically—and maybe even physically—to relieve the pain. I assured her I was okay. She was a sweetheart, asking if I needed a bed to lie down in. I declined, letting her know this was normal for me, like blinking. It had become autonomic. She kept her eyes on me but moved to the other side of the room, which was getting smaller with the arrival of each new person.

Having my son Tim there with me was a boost. He was a rock, at least on the outside. On the inside, I'm sure he was fighting his own battles, but he was the comfort I needed at the time. I gave him comfort back, putting my arm around him and patting his shoulder.

Dr. Belcastro knew about Jim; she called his commander at Camp Lejuene and had him released from military duty to fly back and be with Kyle. Jim's sergeant worked on getting him a leave immediately. It was one of the gifts we were given. Jim wouldn't be able to get there fast enough to say goodbye, but he was on his way. This gesture by Kyle's doctor, added to everything else she did, demonstrated the wonderful human she was. I'm positive she went extra steps for each of her young oncology patients.

Kyle roused from sleep one last time, just long enough to talk to his mother in quiet, personal tones. She held one of his hands and stroked his hair with her fingers. Her eyes were beyond concern, stuck in a deeper place. He told her that his headache was gone, his stomach had stopped hurting, and that he loved her. It was an intensely personal moment between a mother and her son. Then he slipped gently into a coma.

Kyle fell into a deeper coma as his breathing stopped, following his ancestors who had left this life before. The balloons and flowers seemed futile. The clock stopped, with none of us knowing what to do with our tear-filled eyes and shaky hands. The room was silent and empty despite all the people there.

There is a grave and a headstone, where his shell lay next to his grandfather. On it, it reads, "He touched our hearts and changed our lives forever." His name and dates are inscribed above. On the west-facing side of the stone is engraved a set of mountains with a ski boat on a lake and an antlered deer looking on. It is a perfect monument for Kyle, but tombstones are meaningless, at best. Kyle is not there. He is buried deep in our hearts and minds with a powerful memory.

I'll never lose my memories of my son. They are prized possessions. He taught me more than I could have ever taught him.

There is nothing more final than losing a young child. Only those emotionally battered parents who have faced the ordeal can truly understand. There is loss, and then there is the loss of a child—a child you loved and cared for and raised for a limited time until all you are left with are memories.

30

There was a cloudy transition after Kyle's funeral. A void followed us everywhere. We were wounded physically, spiritually, and mentally. The throbbing pain shrunk at times, though never truly disappeared. Nevertheless, our tears subsided, and the pain scabbed over as life shuttled us forward.

Reality hit and I was back at work, making cardiac appointments, doing home improvements, visiting our church, and still holding tight to my chest. Dr. Vandoven ordered a cardiac cardiolite imaging test—more commonly known as a stress test—shortly after Kyle's death and approximately seven months after my heart bypass surgery. I had absolutely no knowledge of cardiolite, though the word has a nice flow to it. It sounds like something you can buy from late night TV ads, involving a blue light and sonic waves to massage your neck. It isn't.

At the time, I had never heard of a stress test for the heart, though I thought I had been through one before. I know what the word *stress* means. I have been married more times than I can count on one hand. Well, that's not true; it just feels that way. But the memories of counting past marriages sometimes weighs down my soul. I wasn't sure what he was talking about, but I knew I had been through my own stress test.

Dr. Vandoven explained it to me. I would run on a treadmill while a nurse injected me with radioactive isotopes. I would be wired to monitors and forced to overwork my heart. I thought I may have seen an episode involving it on the science fiction channel. No problem. I ran a treadmill four days a week at Gold's Gym. I ignored the radioactive part.

When Dr. Vandoven said he had set me up for a stress test in two weeks, I thought little of it. Another test, more blood work, a new technician, a different thumping or growling machine. No one made me fully understand it was literally going to "stress my heart." Those three words sound uncomfortable at best. I didn't know I would be on a treadmill, running uphill with the machine set on get-the-hell-outa-here speed. I would have radioactive isotopes screaming through my veins, monitors beeping, and Nurse Ratched at the helm.

The test began with an IV line inserted in the forearm of your choice. That was the last time I had a choice. The rest was dictated swiftly. After the designated wait, I was led to a room where I lay down on a long cooking tray and was covered with a triple-folded white sheet. I received a pillow for my head, then I was rolled through a large, off-white donut, with my chest centered in the hole of the donut. I grimaced; the pillow was barely softer than a fireplace grate. I was told to keep my arms behind my head, as though being arrested. Another pillow was inserted under my knees. It was a comfortable position to hold for one minute, maybe two. The technician told me the process took about twelve minutes. I knew I was in trouble. Confined, holding the same position for twelve minutes, reclining on a metal tray, trapped by a chest donut, I began taking deep breaths and doing times tables in my head. The image of my still body kept flashing through my mind. The machine wasn't even turned on yet.

The technician wandered around the room and off to a back area as though we had all the time in the world. The tech had the physique of a lumberjack or an eighteenth-century blacksmith. He had scarred arms, a barrel chest, puffy schoolboy cheeks, and hair he was training to go one way while it went the other. He had a low, quiet voice that sounded more like rumbling trucks on a highway than words. I had to tilt my head to hear him.

"Okay, keep still," the tech rumbled. He made sure I was positioned right then moved carefully to a room behind a window.

The machine began a clanking sound. After a long thirty seconds or so, the donut rotated a small fraction. More clanking, another tiny movement, then another. There were no clocks in the room. I was sure an hour had passed, and the blacksmith tech had gone to lunch, or perhaps off shift. I tried stretching my neck between clanks, to see if anyone was there. I decided the stress must be from waiting for the stress test to be over.

The blacksmith came in from a different door. "Only a bit longer," he proclaimed.

I asked, "Are we in the final seconds, or are we still talking minutes? Or . . . hours?"

He responded, "Three more minutes."

"It's only been nine minutes? Your test is working; I have high anxiety."

He smiled. "This isn't the stress part . . . yet."

"That's not real reassuring," I blurted out, holding my body still.

Shooting pain was forming in my arms that I still held uncomfortably above my head. I tried moving my fingers. It hurt more. I twisted my neck slightly, trying to release the stiffness in my shoulders. I wiggled my toes and stretched my calf muscles. My genetics were not put together to strike a pose and hold it. I'm made for constant movement and agility.

Finally, the intermittent clanging stopped. The tech came to the bottom of the tray and slid me out. I was released from bondage. I stood, bouncing on the balls of my feet. I heard joints pop as I did arm stretches and twists. It felt great to be released.

I asked, "Is this image machine okay? It makes a lot of noise. How old is it?"

Spencer answered, "It works fine. It's been going since 1963."

"You realize a new computer lasts only about five years and is outdated in six months?" I asked, nodding my head toward the machine.

Spencer pointed across the hall, saying, "I'll see you back here after the treadmill."

I crinkled my brow. "I do this *again*?"

"Yes, but next time it's shorter—only seven minutes."

There was a lady in the hall waiting for her turn on the tray. She smiled at me, her arm held straight out with IV tubes taped down.

I smiled and pointed back to the room I just left. "I hope you get better music than I did; all I got was clanging."

She looked puzzled. Her mouth opened as if to say something. Finally, she gave me a funny grin, like she had eaten something sour.

Two nurses were waiting for me with serious or bored expressions on their faces—I wasn't sure which. One asked for my name. I replied. She nodded her head as if I got that question right.

The same one asked, "Mr. Huntsman, could you take off your shirt?"

"Yes, would you like that?" I replied.

She smiled—not a full-on grin, more of an acknowledgment. I took off my shirt, unconsciously flexed, then thought better of it as I looked down at the white scar tissue that separated my chest into two halves. I stood patiently while they unwound a rat's nest of wires with colored tips.

The talking one asked, "Have you done this before? Had a stress test?"

"No, but I do like to try everything once."

"Well, good! Then this will go quickly," she responded.

They had me lie back on an exam table while one of the nurses attached adhesive pads with snaps, then wires, to my chest. I gave her my full smile while she attached the last of the adhesive pads to the wires.

The other one asked questions from her clipboard. My answer about my beta blocker startled her. "Yes, I took all my pills," an answer that made her head jerk.

She tried another angle, as if I didn't understand the first time. "You took your Carvedilol this morning?"

"Yes," I paused. "That would be included in all my pills."

"Didn't anyone tell you not to take your beta blocker this morning?"

"No; is that bad?" I was a bit confused.

"Yes."

She turned to the other one, who was busy with the computer in the corner. In a voice that sounded as though she was tattling in a school yard, she said, "Mr. Huntsman took his beta blocker this morning."

"Really, and no one told you not to?"

This was getting old. I glanced at the other nurse as she turned her head. I hadn't been tattled on since my little sister told my mom I had walked in the ladies' restroom at a store. I was only ten years old at the time and hadn't known I was in the wrong bathroom until I heard ladies talking outside my stall. I was so scared I stood on the toilet, holding on to the latch until I heard the voices leave and the door close. Then I ran out, banging the stall door and crashing into racks of clothing. That's where my sister found me. She made a demeaning childhood remark, smacked my arm, laughed, and ran to tell my mom. My mom was wonderful. She said nothing. I was still embarrassed. My sister kept pointing at me and giggling. I replied by pulling faces like any ten-year-old.

I tried to reply to the nurses, explaining like I was that ten-year-old again. I said each word slowly for emphasis. "I wasn't told about my medicine. I was just told not to eat or drink. I took all my pills, including my beta-blocker, Carvedilol."

Both nurses gave an audible sigh. "Okay," said one, "we'll just have to see if we can get the heart up to stress."

That didn't sound good. She made it sound painful and troublesome. Just when I was starting to connect with her, she seemed to have a mean streak.

I had walked in the hospital full of myself, feeling as though I had a totally functioning heart and a pretty sturdy ego. In reality, I knew I had a rebuilt heart with one-third of my cardiac muscle dead as a corpse. I was getting used to walking briskly, thirty minutes a day. I stood erect. But even though I hadn't yet been on this treadmill from hell, I was feeling battle weary. I was feeling like that ten-year-old who had been tattled on. Things had changed.

I was walked to the treadmill, my two nurses guiding my elbow and my electronic wires to the machine. I was hesitant but positive as they helped me as if they were escorting an old lady across a busy street. They obviously thought I could run like a deer on the treadmill but getting over to it was beyond my limits. The two-foot-wide belt of the treadmill began to rotate, and I started my stress trek.

When I exercise at the gym, I set the treadmill flat, with the belt running between two and three miles per hour, the pace of a swift walk. I do that for a half hour with my heart beating like a cat in a sack. For the stress test, they started at five and jammed it quickly toward ten, all the while slowly elevating the front until I gasped for breath. My heart was slamming against my chest as if I was running up the side of an endless cinderblock wall of a Costco. My pulse raced with fear that the machine might explode.

I had never run uphill at the gym, and now I knew why. My tongue tasted like sawdust; my lungs were filled with stale air. The room became hot; sweat sheened my skin. The machine groaned as the belt whirled and whistled. One nurse kept checking my blood pressure. I concentrated on breathing and not falling off the out-of-control machine. It hurt to breathe, but I gasped for more. My hands held the rails in a death grip. The machine roared. Lungs burned. Heart pounded.

Finally, the treadmill began a rapid descent in noise and motion. It leveled off then slowed. I was wheezing and dizzy. It stopped. My legs noodled as I sucked air like a manic shop vac. The nurses eased me on to an exam table and had me sit with my head toward my knees. I prayed that my lungs wouldn't burst.

"We are going to have to let you rest," said one of the nurses. "Then we'll try an injection to stress your heart. Your Carvedilol pills wouldn't let it get to the point we need."

You flippin' want to do this again? I wanted to cry, but breathing was essential, so I waited. I glanced down to make sure my heart hadn't burst through my chest, leaving broken ribs and shredded skin in its wake. It seemed intact. I said a short prayer. A headache throbbed as my brain bellowed for air.

Time passed quietly and slowly. The nurses wandered off, probably for coffee and a giggle. I looked around at gray wallpaper and white ceiling squares. Colored wires flowed down off my chest, pooling on the sheet beside me. My breathing returned to normal, my skin changed from sweaty crimson to its normal pink, and my legs lay flaccid without bone or structure.

Centuries passed before the nurses came back, but they appeared refreshed and ready for another go at me. I searched my brain for bravery but found only a stew of fear. My blood pressure was taken from the cuff that dangled from my arm. They reattached the wires to the machine. I was laid back on the exam table with my back raised about sixty degrees. It was short-term comfortable. They explained that I would feel my heart race, but when it got to a certain point, another drug would be injected to lower my heart rate. Simple, right?

My heart was pounding within a second after the injection. My mouth widened. I think my tongue hung out over my lower lip, and my eyes bulged outside my eyelids. My chest was in torture. I leaned back, sucking air through my lips like a fish flopping on a boat deck. I was dizzy, miserable, frightened, and confused, and I wondered how long I might live. I truly hated these nurses. They were both Doctor Mengele in drag.

"That's it!" I heard.

The other drug was injected into my IV line. My heart put on its brakes. My body quivered. I pulled slow, grand breaths into my lungs and held my chest as the pain slowly subsided. I lay back down, lightheaded, waiting for the aftereffects to wear down.

It was like ending a really bad date; I couldn't get out of that room and away from those two sadistic nurses fast enough. I waited in the hall for my turn with the radiologist. It came quickly.

I was back on the tray, pulled through the donut with my hands in the air behind me, centered just so, and told to relax for a few minutes. I was cold, so he brought me a thin warmed blanket. There was much better service in his room. I should have tipped him.

The donut machine began clanging every so often and doing that timed tortoise movement, clockwise. I was exhausted from nurse torture, so it was easy to lie still the second time. I had almost fallen asleep when he nudged me and said, "We're done."

Pulling my arms from behind my head, I found they had gone to sleep. I had that sharp needle pain going up and down my arm muscles. The joints wouldn't bend right. It hurt to lift myself up from the tray.

I *thanked* the technician and walked wearily out the two doors to the hall. There was still tingling in my arms, though it was not painful, just annoying. I drove home, feeling exhausted. I slept for hours. I couldn't remember arriving home and hoped I hadn't hit anything.

Since then I have had the stress test three other times. The first time was the only bad one, because my prescription meds kept my heart beating slowly. With the others, I didn't take my beta blocker or any of my other medications until after the test. So those tests went as smoothly as could be.

I will never see a heart stress test as a good thing. The difficulty of my first time was an anomaly, but it's hard to go back for something so unpleasant, especially as your memory embellishes it. There is something about taking an impaired heart muscle to its limits to test how that affects it and get a reading that seems completely out of whack.

The test does measure your ejection fraction, which allows the doctor to give estimations on how long your heart will keep pumping, how healthy you will be in the future, and where you stand in the statistics of normal versus diseased. Also, it helps the doctor identify improvements and deteriorations in heart performance. It helps the doctor identify which medications could work for you. It is also a test I should have had prior to my heart attack. But if that had been done, I'd have nothing to write about.

31

My health stabilized. I discovered a working point where I didn't overdo it. I learned to stay away from things that caused shortness of breath and angina. I developed a rhythm with my daily activities and exercise. It wasn't perfect, but it was workable.

With the help of my sons, we began building a cabin from the foundation up on farm property in the middle of Utah, overlooking the tail end of Yuba Lake. The land had been in Diana's family through decades of sheep and cattle ranching. We had purchased a thirteen-acre parcel of it for our newest adventure. It was a two-hour drive from our home in Salt Lake—an hour and a half if my wife drove.

I was fairly adept at home improvement projects. Having completed previous rentals and unfinished basements, I had an idea about framing and sixteen-inch centers. I armed myself with Band-Aids and Neosporin for cuts and several pairs of tweezers to remove the slivers of wood that always seemed to become installed in my fingers. I have power tools—a radial arm saw, a table saw, a compressor and nail guns, and a circular saw. I've also accumulated hammers, chisels, levels, and the knowledge to keep my fingers away from moving blades. I'm also great at picking up how-to-books from the library and studying them until I get the general concept. It's not a perfect construction system, but what I lack in knowledge, I make up for in spirit. I also know how to swear, throw tools down, and redo a project. And, to paraphrase, "I am a man that knows my limitations," as Clint Eastwood put it in *Dirty Harry*. I am also stubborn enough to have few. I was set.

Diana has helped me many times through renovations. She thinks she knows more than she does, but as a farm girl, she is adept at more than I'd ever admit. Two of our boys, Jim and

Tim, worked construction, so their knowledge and help were invaluable. Our oldest, Jeremy, follows directions well and has learned enough about construction in the process to be a big help. Together we made a pretty good work crew, though at times it was the blind, deaf, dumb, and haughty leading the blind, deaf, dumb, and haughty. It's hard to put that many Type A personalities together and not have a workforce of bosses. We were bosses that love each other, nonetheless.

The foundation was professionally poured for a basement with eight-foot ceilings. Moving cement around, in any capacity, did not seem heart healthy. There are the can do's and the will not do's. Pouring cement and moving the heavy sludge was a definite will not do.

Diana, my sons, and I laid the floor joists and the sub-floor. We constructed and raised the two-by-six studded walls. Windows were set precariously without having to use one Band-Aid. A view was created and admired. We laid out the loft and hammered joists into place, taking up about half the length of the cabin. This took a couple of weekends.

The main roof beam that ran from fore to aft gave us some trouble. The east- and west-facing walls were cut out to fit the five-by-sixteen-inch beam. We tried for about an hour to lower the beam into place. It would bind, slipping into one side and not the other. Jeremy hung down from one end of the beam with legs and arms wrapped around it, looking like a gorilla hanging off a limb. His body jerked up and down as he tried to force the end into the slot. He tried sitting on top, his butt bouncing heavily on the beam. He tried other positions, all precarious, all simian. None of his attempts worked—and all were quite dangerous.

The beam hung almost thirty feet in the air off a telescoping forklift. The wind blew just enough to kick dust up from time to time. The sun reddened the back of our necks while I maneuvered the arm on the enormous blue forklift, trying to judge my target. My sons let me know that what I was doing was wrong each time. I tried to appreciate their help. I didn't. We re-measured the beam and the cutout. It should fit, we concluded. After several stretch and beer breaks, I moved the stick a touch up, then gently down. The main beam dropped into position with ease and perfection. Sometimes taking a break from a project helps solve it. Certainly, cursing hadn't worked.

The metal hangers were spaced evenly, the I-beams inserted and power-nailed in. The boys started to put up the roofing plywood, but the wind had kicked up. A rainstorm was forming and looked inevitable. Every so often the wind would grab a sheet from their hands and sail it forty feet away. Flying plywood is hazardous in many ways, so we quit building for the weekend. It was fine with me; my heart was over-taxed. My lungs seemed ready to collapse. The rain came down—perfectly refreshing. The smell of wet leaves and branches dripping their perfume, mixed with soaked sagebrush, was unforgettable.

The next weekend we met again on a Friday night. We sat around the campfire exchanging stories and downing beverages. The boys preferred pop-top cans of beer and voices that grew louder as the garbage sack of aluminum cans filled. I was on my heart-healthy single glass of red wine that I sipped through the starlit night. Diana enjoyed a vanilla Coke. All my boys were there; Jeremy and Tim came down together, and Jim arrived late that night from Portland.

On those campfire nights, I wore out and hit the bed about midnight. Diana usually put in an extra hour or two before seeking me in the motor home. The boys called it a night not too far from sunrise, about four or five in the morning. This would be their tradition for years to come. Someday in the future they will be realistic and mature, like their father, but for now, five a.m. is their weekend bedtime. Anything before that is party time.

I remember those days—able to stay up all hours of the night, grab a couple of winks of sleep, and show up to work in rough shape but ready to go, then getting home and passing out on the couch until ten. Waking up and doing it all over again. The sweet days of youth. At the time, I assumed that energy would never end. What is that saying about youth being wasted on the young?

I was always the first one up, by choice. My internal camping alarm went off about six a.m. I restarted the fire and complained to myself about all the empty beer cans, everywhere but in the trash. I made a big breakfast of hash browns, scrambled eggs, sliced ham, and toast. I ate by myself in front of the fire, reading a book in the morning solitude. It was always a nice, quiet time filled with contemplation and memorable sunrises, with morning birds filling the silence with their happy trilling.

I ended my relaxation planning the day in my head. It didn't always go the way I figured. Sometimes I took that in stride; other times, not so much. Heart failure had made me more scheduled and less easygoing. I got irritated at angina and things I couldn't control.

I did a few morning cleaning duties. The food I made for everyone else was wrapped up in tin foil, ready for when they woke up. My paper plate and plastic spoon went into the fire. I was ready to work.

The food waited at least three hours, but usually longer, for the rest of the family crew. Sometimes they ate it. Other times they peered under the tin foil and crinkled their noses. It *had* been sitting a while. Flies were trying to get at it. Diana always had cereal and milk.

It was the same old stuff every trip. I assumed they wanted to get an early start. My mind couldn't wrap around the fact they were in their late teens and early twenties. For them, Saturday mornings arrived at noon.

Even with a bad heart, I was a workaholic. I started the generator and hooked up the nail gun as the sun rose and cast long shadows. I knew they would get up when they got up. It was invigorating to exercise my heart and see projects develop. I paced my tasks; if I didn't, I ended up on Tylenol and bedsheets by noon.

The weekends after were clear and filled with sunscreen. Slowly, the cabin took shape. The inside was finished to a point of tentative residency. I bought a queen-sized bed for the main bedroom. Split logs were nailed to the outside and stained. A stove, gas fireplace heater, and propane fridge were installed. The large porch was finished with round wooden rails. A bathroom was roughed in for the day when our outhouse would be closed.

My heart seemed to keep up with all that work quite well. In fact, it seemed to improve with the exercise and psychological fulfillment. I still wasn't scaling up and down ladders or lifting boulders, but my stamina grew. I believe the heart rejuvenates in its own way. Heart muscle lost is always gone, but I believe you can strengthen and refine what cardiac muscle you still have.

We still visit our cabin most weekends through the warm months. The "to do" list never ends, though our time working on it has dropped considerably. It's nice to have a place of solitude, away from the anxiety of work, bills, and noise. There is restful peacefulness in sitting around a campfire with family and friends, enjoying conversation and bright constellations. We have no television to glue us to a couch at night. We boat during the day and enjoy the late nights. It is a place to exercise my heart muscle and to let it rest in an open-space peacefulness that is hard to explain.

32

My health went mostly up, but sometimes down, over the next few years as I lived life like a tattered, overused umbrella. Sometimes I was fully open; other times, I sat upright in a corner of uselessness, without any signs of life. I was mostly that open umbrella, shedding the rain. But there were always those times of stormy weather and rain pelting down, when I remained unopened.

When my ejection fraction dropped, the umbrella closed. I became lethargic and dizzy. For me, lethargy means having to sit down after minimal exercise, such as a walk. It hurt to breathe. Oxygen came in short gasps. After a brief period of about five to ten minutes, I would regain my normal breathing, angina would evaporate, and I could stand without my eyes rolling back in my head like a slot machine after a hard pull.

For a person with coronary disease, knowing your ejection fraction is a must. It is not something they check all that often, but heart patients follow it religiously. If you look up the definition in a medical book, *ejection fraction* (EF) is a bit muddy. It would take at least two years of medical school, comprehension of a scientific calculator, third-year college algebra, and an understanding of fluid dynamics to follow its formal definition.

But it is quite simple once you understand a few basics about how the heart works. Your heart circulates blood through two separate pumps that force blood from one place to another, like squeezing water out of a water balloon by compressing it in your hand. Except there are four balloons, two on the top and two on the bottom. The two on top (atriums) receive the blood. The two on the bottom (ventricles) are the pumps. Your left pump (ventricle) forces oxygen-rich blood throughout your body through your arteries. Oxygen-depleted blood returns to the top right receiving dock (atrium) and passes it down to the right pump (ventricle). The right pump (ventricle) pumps this blood to the lungs to pick up oxygen, then returns it to the top left receiving dock (atrium). From there, it is passed to the bottom left pump (ventricle), which again forces oxygen-rich blood throughout your body. This cycle goes continuously, whether you are sleeping, playing golf, doing dishes, having sex, mowing the lawn, arguing with the neighbors, climbing a tree, or nesting on the couch in front of an endless drool of flat-screen sitcoms.

Back to ejection fraction. As I mentioned, when the left pump (ventricle) contracts, it ejects oxygen-carrying blood out into the body through the arteries. It is the bigger pump of the two, has the largest chamber, and is where heart function is measured. This is the ejection part.

The fraction part happens because no matter how hard your heart muscle works to squeeze out as much blood as possible, some blood remains in the chamber, waiting for the next contraction. The amount the left ventricle pumps out per beat out of the total amount in its chamber is referred to as the "ejection fraction." So, there is always an amount that is not pumped. Ideally, more is pumped out than left behind.

A normal ejection fraction is about 50 to 70 percent. That's where most healthy people are at. If you are at 40 percent, there could be a heart problem. If you have an EF below 30 percent, you definitely have a cardiac problem. Somewhere around 20 and below indicates a serious problem.

My EF stayed at about 35 percent after my heart attack. With exercise and pharmaceutical therapy, I was trying to nudge it up a bit. Many years after my bypass surgery, my ejection fraction dropped down to 19. Alarms went off.

Dr. Vandoven changed my medicines slightly. He decided to recheck me in sixty days, instead of the normal six months.

My wife went into research mode, becoming hell-bent on me getting a heart transplant. Whole trees came out of our printer as she amassed stifling information about transplants. She spent sleepless nights doing computer research. Surgical and hospital data grew like a paper flower garden throughout our condo. Stacks that I should read. Stacks that she needed to get back to.

Stacks of medical gibberish with yellow, red, and blue 3-M stickers jutting out with scribbles on each one. Stacks of yellow-highlighted information and plastic garbage liners filled with crumpled sheets of paper. She almost had her own cardiac infarction when the ink cartridge dried up and shriveled inside the printer, which then began whistling smoke out the sides. Her process came from love. We decorated our home in notepads and paper.

I was of the mindset that I could get back to normal with naps and a little work on a treadmill. My whole life, I have felt that a good, positive attitude and a shower can heal most anything. My mom believed in tea and toast as the cure-all. My plan worked for me. I also believed my cardiologist would come up with an idea or two. He usually did.

Several days later, I got a call from Dr. Vandoven's nurse Rachael to set an appointment in two weeks. My cardiologist wanted to go over a few alternatives. He had heard from my wife about the transplant idea. I was pretty sure he intended to head that one off.

Two weeks passed. I had an afternoon cardiologist appointment shortly after a blood test. I waited my allotted time in the reception area. I watched the fish in the tank instead of reading the battered magazines. The nurse escorted me through the standard routine—weight, blood pressure, oxygen level.

I've mentioned before that besides congestive heart failure, I have Reynaud's phenomenon. On cold days, it allows a minimal amount of circulation in my hands and fingers, making the oxygen test useless—and it's been hell on snow skiing days. The nurse was having trouble getting my oxygen number. I rubbed my hands together and blew hot breath on my fingertips. I moved the clip to another finger and finally got a reading—97 percent. The green-eyed nurse was happy, and we moved down the hall to a room. In the room, she went through my list of medications. This was routine, and I knew the nurse would get a scolding if Dr. Vandoven found out she didn't ask.

I turned to the nurse as she put the blood pressure cuff around my arm. "I haven't been in this room before. This is a big exam room. This must be the luxury suite of exam rooms."

She replied, "Yeah, most of them are pretty small. Three people and it's crowded."

"So, I have been upgraded? Is there an extra charge to my insurance?"

She giggled while taking off the BP cuff. "No. This is a perk for being a good patient."

"I have been a patient of Dr. Vandoven for so many years," I said, "I'm sure I've paid for this room several times over."

My nurse smiled as she exited.

Before she closed the door, I asked, "Can I request this room next time? Is there a waiting list?"

All I saw was her hand wave at me as she shut the door.

I turned to Diana, who was sitting quietly in a corner chair. It was unusual and nice to have her join me for one of my appointments. I had someone to talk to. "For a suite, they should have better pictures. Though, you've got to love the color on that poster of the dissected heart. A masterpiece of realism art."

She was texting and ignored me.

"Just look at the expressive lines over there. The up-and-down stroke of the heart rhythms. It takes your breath away."

I was still being ignored. To a child in his fifties, this became a contest, a game, a search for the win. I was not easily tuned out and avoided. I leaned over her, flapping my palms in front of her face. "Hello . . . helloooooo, lady in a text coma. Hello!"

She hit my belly softly with the back of her hand. A devilish smile conjured up.

"I'm seeing small amounts of life in that chair. I believe it may be my wife, holding a rectangular plastic God in her hand. Her fingers are fluttering, as if communicating somehow. I think her essence is being sucked into the cell phone, one letter at a time."

Diana finally looked up. "Just sit down. How old are you?"

"Fifty-plus, going on eight and a half."

She retorted, "Eight is giving you the benefit of the doubt." She crinkled her nose up and flipped me off.

"Oh, oh . . . real mature," I responded.

She burst into a deep-down laugh. "Well, what about this?" She began shaking her palms in front of my face, mimicking me.

"I was trying to get your attention."

"So you could explain your take on the artwork in the room? I was listening. I just refused to comment and join the world of a five-year-old."

"You know this Jef-bashing is hard on my cardiac persona," I said sarcastically as I held both hands over my left chest, bowed over slightly, and performed the tiniest of whines.

She shook her head and started to say something. She was interrupted by the door swinging open. A smiling Dr. Vandoven entered with a small laptop in his arms. After the greetings and the mandatory how-do-you-feel question-and-answer period, he sat down on the remaining chair and faced us.

My cardiologist has a way of talking intellectually to his patients. He doesn't talk down to us. He explains, using those wonderful words of knowledge and concern. I have always hated physicians who try to explain maladies as though I have the intellect of a box elder tree. I have been conversing in English for a long time—more than fifty years. I resent being talked to in one- and two-syllable words, as if it's my first day of kindergarten and I'm listening to an explanation of how to drink my milk and take a nap.

Dr. Vandoven got right to the meat of our visit. He had decided I needed an acronym for my heart—an ICD. I was leery of all acronyms but listened with trepidation. He went over his reasons for wanting me to have an implantable cardioverter defibrillator—an ICD, more commonly known as a pacemaker— placed in my chest. The main purpose of an ICD was to adjust heart rhythm.

New treatments never sound good, acronym or not.

He explained that the lower chambers of my heart (ventricles) were not pumping in sync with the upper chambers (atria). This meant the left ventricle could not pump enough blood to my body. He said that eventually this would lead to more heart failure symptoms, such as shortness of breath, fatigue, and rapid or irregular heartbeat. The ICD would be imbedded in my upper chest with tiny wire leads implanted through veins into specific places in my heart. The leads would send small electrical impulses to help my heart beat in a more balanced way. Dr. Vandoven said this therapy would decrease the symptoms of heart failure, improve the quality of my life, and hopefully raise my ejection fraction.

Having something implanted in my chest sounded painful in so many ways. But I was optimistic, and I trusted that my doctor knew something about the procedure and the necessity.

We were shown color, fold-over charts and diagrams of the ICD and the heart. Dr. Vandoven pointed out all the positive attributes of the technology. It would come with a built-in defibrillator in case my heart stopped. *Uhhh . . . wait . . . my heart stopping? My heart might stop, as in cease?* He also mentioned the negatives, as if a stopped heart wasn't negative enough—such as the slight possibility of infection and a short five- to seven-year battery life. The positives definitely outweighed any negatives in my mind. I was relieved. This was much better than a transplant.

My last occupation had been as a buyer and manager of retail electronics, so I was also thinking the implantation of an electronic device sounded morbidly cool. If Hitachi or Kenwood made ICDs, perhaps I could get a discount. Maybe they could even incorporate an iPod into it, with extra leads to my auditory canals. Just a thought; I really would enjoy some music.

Diana nodded "yes" for both of us. I was still concerned about the stopped heart thing.

The implantation was scheduled for three weeks later with a surgeon named Dr. Tysdale. It seems my insurance would only cover certain surgical hospitals. Dr. Vandoven did not have surgical privileges where my insurance would allow my surgery. He was annoyed but said Dr. Tysdale was incredible at the procedure and that he had done hundreds of them. *Whew!*

I met my new surgeon a few days prior to the implant. He was chubby-faced and jovial. Dr. Tysdale had on a lab coat with his name stitched in blue above the pocket. He had rounded, sturdy shoulders and the movements of someone at ease with himself, effervescent with accompanying hand gestures. His happy nature, disheveled hair, and empathy made me instantly like the man. He explained the procedure with a smile.

During our visit, Dr. Tysdale's nurse called him out into the hall. When he came back, he was almost giddy. In an excited voice, he explained that he had great news. Essentially, my heart was just bad enough to receive a biventricular pacemaker. *Whatever that was.* He seemed quite happy about this. We returned the smile. Even so, it seemed strange to be ecstatic over the news of having a battery-operated, metallic device inserted in my chest and connected by tiny wires to my heart. He explained that the good news meant that I would receive three leads instead of the normal two. We became excited because he was excited. *I was going to have three leads and an implantable battery device surgically placed in my chest. And I would have a defibrillator in the pacemaker to shock me to the floor if my heart went out of whack. Oh, happy day!*

Diana is the practical one on this type of stuff. The attorney side of her comes out. She asked about the three leads and why they were better than two. She dissolved the contagious giddiness I had caught from the doctor, and I became suspicious about this ominous device.

Dr. Tysdale joked about more always being better. Then he talked about AV synchrony. It seems the third lead in a biventricular ICD helps the left ventricle contract at the same time as the right ventricle. It paces two different parts of the heart, for better force, so one part is not lagging behind. The two ventricles working together pump more blood with greater efficiency. More blood means more oxygen to the cells of my body. So, I should feel better, overall.

I was all for that. I signed the paperwork for the implant adventure. I was psyched, but I knew that as soon as I got home from the appointment reality would hit, with anxiety close on its heels. I kept looking at my upper chest and thinking about surgically slipping something the size of a cell phone into my chest and running wires to my heart, as though I was a radio being repaired. The whole plan seemed a bit Terminator crazy to me. I looked down at my cell phone, then pushed my fingers against my upper chest. *There isn't a lot of meat there.*

Then, the permanently installed defibrillator came to mind. I recalled those paddles from defibrillators on hospital shows, with the body bouncing up from the bed. That didn't sound at all good. Fear surfaced.

"I am having something inserted under my skin that can shock my heart with a strong force." I took in a big, long breath of air and signed papers saying it was what I wanted. *Hmmm?*

We arrived at the Intermountain Medical Center on January 4, 2008, eight years after my bypass surgery. Diana wanted to drop my fifty-six-year-old body off at the front door so I wouldn't have to walk from the parking lot. I walked from parking lots all the time. I could certainly walk from this one. We argued. She won. I got out at the front door. I asked if she could just hold my hand through the automatic doors, perhaps find me a wheelchair, so I wouldn't have to put one leg in front of the other too many times? She shooed me out of the vehicle with a few expletives and a slap on my rear. As her car pulled away, Diana pointed an index finger at me like a gun.

I hate being pampered. There is something truly annoying about it when it is not needed. I mumbled to myself, "When I need a wheelchair or help to the couch, I'll ask for it." Like a lost puppy, I walked the short distance to the front door as I had been told and waited for her. Is obedience part of the marriage vows?

Because I would be getting anesthesia, I had not been allowed to eat or drink that morning. I had brushed my teeth and swished water around in my mouth, then spat it out. I was thirsty and hungry. I licked my teeth hoping for nourishment—nothing good. A flavor like citrus cleaning solvent hung in my mouth. I found a drinking fountain and let the water flow across my outstretched tongue, willing myself not to take a gulp. Nothing helped. My throat cracked and dried like a Mojavi noon.

The surgical sign-in area graced rows of chairs, a busy young lady with glasses edged on her nose sitting behind a computer screen, plastic barrels, and the sound of water dripping. Blue buckets and plastic garbage cans sat around the check-in area like sentries standing post. Water from above was dripping briskly into each one. Plunk . . . plunk . . . plunk!

We maneuvered through the cans as our eyes scanned the thirty-foot ceiling. The receptionist twirled her upraised finger around, saying, "We have a leak upstairs." With that master-of the-obvious announcement, she began asking us questions and typing our answers into the computer. She copied my insurance cards, printed out pages for me to sign, and asked us to wait. We were back in a waiting room again, but at least it was dripping.

The place looked like the makings of a disaster area. Caution tape was wrapped around support pillars. I watched as the water beaded up, ran the length of a white ceiling beam, and plunked steadily into a thirty-gallon tub within a few feet of us. A hospital maintenance man changed out the full garbage pails that were catching more of a stream than a drip. He looked worried as he glanced up. The ambiance of the place needed a little work. I wondered about the integrity of the roof above and slid our chairs under a support beam.

I tried to read my book, but the dripping kept drawing me in. I set my book down and leaned toward Diana, saying, "I've never been to this hospital before, and this is not a great first impression."

She smiled.

"I hope that," I pointed to the roof, "is not coming from the OR."

Diana looked at me. "No, that wouldn't be a good thing."

"Yeah, it would get everyone's foot booties all wet. You think they are slipping and sliding up there, trying to do a bowel resection or a boob job? Like working in the shower." I was finding humor in this catastrophe, as usual.

"I just hope whatever is up there doesn't come down here, full force," Diana giggled. She dropped her shoulders, clamped her hands, and gazed up praying.

"Uh oh," I said, "did you hear that? . . . It *is* the OR. I just heard someone say, 'oops.' I think we'd better leave while we can. Maybe we should come back on a different day. Preferably, one where the rain is outside instead of inside the lobby."

A lady in blue sporting a stethoscope necklace began staring at me and approached. She said, "Mr. Huntsman?" I hesitated, still watching the dripping water, somewhat mesmerized. She signaled, come here, with two fingers. I clasped Diana's hand, and we stood up.

I asked the nurse what was above us. She said they were patient rooms. It seems one of the toilets had overflowed and was leaking. She acted as though it was nothing out of the ordinary. That didn't make me feel any better. Both Diana and I scrunched up our faces in disgust.

Diana questioned her on the proximity of the operating room. We found out it was on the other end of the building and above the leak.

The nurse led us down several corridors and into the prep room. My new outfit for the next few hours was on the bed. I was told I could keep on my own underwear. With the open back on these gowns, that was more than fine with me.

A prep nurse came in. She shaved my chest, took vitals, hooked me up to an IV, then drew blood from the line. My wait was short. I wasn't even able to crack open a book or check out the news on TV. I was on a gurney kissing my wife goodbye within fifteen minutes. Diana mouthed "Good luck" as I headed down the hallway.

The intravenous sedation was taking hold as I exited an elevator and headed through the double doors, feet first. The dripping was forgotten. My fears from before were gone. It was just another walk at the mall. No, I hate shopping. It was another hike in the mountains. I forgot about the defibrillator shocking me senseless and about implantable cell phones. I was ready. Drugs set my mind at ease.

I woke up groggy, with little feeling under my gauze-wrapped left shoulder. Diana was waiting by my side. Things were blurry—more black-and-white than colored. A nurse attended to the monitor. I was done. I would have a stronger and more precise heartbeat—in the words of the surgeon, "AV synchrony."

Dr. Tysdale entered the room abruptly. I was semi-alert. He asked no one in particular, "How are you doing?" It seemed rhetorical, so I didn't answer. Dr. Tysdale told me everything had gone well. They had tested the device, and everything was working as it should. I would stay overnight in the hospital and probably be released by noon the next day.

I spent an exhausting, uneventful night in the hospital. Again, surgery is debilitating. I didn't read. I didn't watch TV. If I ate at all, I don't remember. I'm always hungry, so I assume I did. I also assume that the food I don't remember was great and the beverages superb.

I was discharged with a few days' worth of Keflex antibiotics and Darvocet for pain. I was scheduled for a two-week checkup on my incision, leaving my hospital bed to another suffering soul. I was lucky enough to go home where I could enjoy my sore chest in peace.

I quit the pain pills after the first day. They tend to burn my insides after a couple of days, much like swallowing battery acid. They also make me loopy, which feels like being dumb-as-dirt. I've always hated that. The pills cause me more pain than they alleviate. I would much rather suffer than be stupid with my stomach lining turning to fire-melting mush.

The chest scar began to heal, peeling off tiny brown clusters of scab in a line. My stamina increased. I still wasn't a ladder climber, but stairs were a cinch. My angina decreased, and my breathing appeared fuller. Not only that, but the shape of my chest changed.

The ICD really looked like an imbedded cell phone in my upper chest, just as I had envisioned. A very expensive cell phone. It costs well over $100,000 to have this one-sided boob-job. I weigh 160 pounds—thin, mostly muscle and bone. I could feel the rippled edges of the ICD, its shape, and the wires coming out at the top left. It was inserted under the skin on top of ribs and muscle. I have little fat, if any, above my pecs to hide the device, so it was a prominent, semi-square, protruding growth. It stuck out almost half an inch above my normal skin level. My grandkids poked it, fascinated, asking me when my "owie" would go away.

It eventually became unnoticeable to me, though moms and children at the condo pool glanced at it often. Now I occasionally find myself wishing I had more fat on my body. *Nah, I'll stay thin.*

When it was first installed, my ICD gave me a kind of rubbing pain, as if it was sliding around in there. Red skin was infected around the right perimeter of the ICD. My cardiologist talked about removing the device, thinking my body was rejecting it. With antibiotics and time, it eventually healed. It has become a familiar, odd, rectangular bump above and to the left of my heart.

Now that I have felt and seen the improvement of my heart, I believe the pacemaker is one of the greatest miracles of science to come out in my lifetime. It was invented before my time—in 1950—but that first external pacemaker and the ICD I have are miles apart. Thank God for that, as well as the scientific and medical teams that have worked on it to make it what it is today. And people say there are no miracles. I say God works with scientists.

Diana asked me the other day how my body was dealing with the pacemaker/ defibrillator. I said, "It has been great. Since they implanted my IUD, there is ominous security about it."

"You mean ICD, don't you?" she replied, laughing. "There is somewhat of a difference between the two."

"Yeah, ICD, that's what I said. An IUD is inserted in a completely different place." I laughed. "You must be mixing the two up."

I got punched in the arm. "Don't play dumb like a fox with me!"

My biventricular ICD gets checked every six months. It allows me to bypass airport and federal building scanners, sent to the side and felt up by latex-gloved men as I stand there, humiliated, in stocking feet and my belt in my hand. We have to arrive early, because this pat-down takes much more time.

Every few months they test my implant. The annoying part is that my heartbeat can be varied with the ease of a computerized machine on a cart and a few key punches. It can race my heart as though I've run a hard mile. The machine can also slow my heart down to a point of almost putting me to sleep. I find that disconcerting, and I hope my wife never buys one on Amazon.

Racing my heart is great, when I'm the one doing it—such as when I move quickly up the stairs to the next floor or run on a treadmill at the gym. When a tech runs the machine and manipulates the beat up and down like a yo-yo, I truly hate it.

There is something completely unnatural about it. The testing does let my cardiologist know how my heart reacts. That is a wonderful thing. It also indicates ways to fine-tune the ICD as my heart changes.

A note about the *D* (defibrillator) in ICD. I keep remembering the dog collar my neighbor's young children used. I recall watching in anger as their dog yelped and shuddered when being followed around the yard by those children, remote in hand. I yelled at the sadistic little kids whenever I saw it happening, which decreased the dog's torture while I was home. Who knows what happened after we moved? That poor animal was a psychiatric mess, in need of a good canine counselor and a new family.

I certainly hope Diana doesn't ever get a remote for my ICD. I would be doing her nails and rubbing her feet every night.

Over the years there have been two instances when the defibrillator part of my ICD has gone off. The first time it happened, I was in Coeur d'Alene, Idaho, a city on a picturesque, pine-surrounded lake not far from the Canadian border.

Diana and I rented a ski boat to spend the day with my son Jim on the lake. The single hull parted the waters as we as we cruised across the main bay. After we toured for an hour or so and played on a small beach, we found a smaller, calmer bay. I wanted to slalom ski, something I hadn't done since my heart attack years earlier. There was a time when I was pretty good at skimming across the water on one ski, leaning way in, fanning a rooster tail high into the sky, and crossing behind the boat to sail over the wake in a polished jump. I assumed I could still do that––like riding a bike.

Since it was chilly mountain water, I donned my wetsuit with tender giddiness. I eased over the edge with one foot in the rubber boot and splashed into the water. I gasped as my head pivoted, checking for ice cubes that I was positive were floating nearby.

It took a minute to get used to the semi-frigid water. I grabbed the end of the tow rope and told Jim to ease the boat out. Soon, the rope tightened. Arms braced straight out. My knees were bent and ready. I yelled, "Hit it." The boat took off. Within seconds, my brain scanned a problem. I threw the rope in the air, releasing it. I had forgotten my life jacket. Oops. They circled back around, and I waved them closer. I handed up the ski and climbed the ladder into the boat.

I toweled off and warmed up. Then I slipped the necessary life jacket over my wet suit. I jumped back into the cold waters. The boat moved slowly away, and the rope tightened. I got into my stance again—muscles tightened in anticipation.

"Hit it!"

The motor roared, the bow lifted as if climbing out, and a massive gurgle of turbulence stirred by the double prop. The rope skimmed the water as it lined itself up straight and taut. I concentrated. My arms were outstretched, my leg muscles bent and ready for the pull, and I leaned slightly back. My arms yanked as the 265-horsepower engine roared. Every muscle in my body tightened. The single ski braced against the weight of water as liquid furrowed in front of me.

I knew immediately something was wrong. The boat wasn't going fast enough. The prop wasn't all the way down. I noticed the boat angled with the front raised high toward the sun—too much angle and not enough speed. I tightened my grip on the handle of the rope and leaned further back, hoping it would pop me to the surface. The ski plowed. Lake water formed a wall on both sides of me, racing and splashing into my face. The momentum of the boat was enough to drag me like an escaped anchor but not enough to cause the lift needed. My muscles exploded.

My breath stopped. My muscles turned flaccid. My body went limp. The boat purred. The rope flipped into the sky. Everything went black. Life stopped.

Electricity surged through my body. The brightness of the day shocked me as my head lifted from beneath the water. My mouth coughed up foul water. I was dazed. My mind struggled to figure out where I was. A wave sloshed over me, and I felt the security of the life jacket that bunched up above my shoulders and lifted at the armpits. Seconds passed and I realized I was in the water. My bare feet dangled below me. Another wave hit and moved on. The ski bumped my shoulder, and I draped my arms over it like a dear friend. My chin rested on the rubber boot.

As I bobbed in the water, I gazed around. The boat was out of sight. The shore lay miles away. Panic raced through my mind. My blood pressure surged. I tried to lift myself up, kicking my legs frantically. Finally, I caught a glimpse of the boat heading my way. I laid back, resting my head on the life jacket, arms wrapped over the ski, exhaustion deep in my icy bones.

They helped me into the boat. Under a mass of towels, I curled into the seat, shivered, and gave a prayer of thanks.

A wonderful thing happened out there in the frigid mountain waters of Lake Coeur d'Alene. I had had a full-fledged cardiac arrest—my heart stopped. Yeah, there's that. But the big thing that happened was it wasn't my time. Something or someone intervened—God, the Source, Jehovah, Elohim, Allah, Abba, the omnipresent creator, or whatever you may call Him or Her.

If what happened took place the first time I had jumped in the water, that time without a life jacket on, I certainly would have drowned. After all the exertion of trying to get up on that water ski and then having my cardiac defibrillator go off (which, trust me, sucks every ounce of energy from you), I wouldn't have been able to hold myself out of the water. I would have bobbed like a lifeless cork, face down.

Sure, I was lucky, but someone added that luck. Someone wanted me to stick around for another day. There have been three times in my life where I should have died. The second two involved my heart stopping, and then by the grace of a higher power my life was given to me again. I'm not a "praise the Lord" kind of person, but I know within the deepest pores of my soul that I was given a second and third and fourth chance. Not sure why. Certainly, I don't believe I'm worth all that much. But I cross my fingers and hope it keeps happening.

33

Life puts weeds in your garden. It's up to you whether you let them flourish and take over where healthy vegetables once grew, or you pull them out. If you only snip off the tops, they will grow heartier and spread. Maintenance is a lot of work, but you need to dig deep and pull out the root. Sure, the seeds of weeds will always follow the wind and resettle on your ground. They are constant. They never go away. You can only deter them; but if you let them go, they take over, and the good plants have the life sucked out of them. That is true living.

There will always be heart maladies and brain tumors and hundreds of other terrible things that can infect our bodies. Only determined action will keep them to a minimum. Just like pulling weeds, you need to eat right, exercise, quit smoking, avoid drugs and alcohol, get to a decent stabilized weight, have regular medical checkups, and then cross your fingers. It is the same with all physical and mental health problems. Nothing is easy. There is satisfaction in having stubbornness and not giving up. Think of these deep-rooted illnesses as only weeds. You, as the patient, must be the gardener. Ignore them or look at them as some ominous force, and they will root deeper and perhaps even take over.

I keep my smiling weed-whacker on high, with a full tank of pre-mixed gas. I try to face each day with the idea of being as healthy as I can. I don't always succeed; sometimes my heart has other ideas, but I still try to guide it.

Daylight comes in through my bedroom window each morning. The couch is comfortable and absorbing, but laps in the pool feel better. Medium-rare steaks smell good on the barbeque, but too many wear my body down. We all have whims and urges at times for the taste or smell of something missing. Sometimes, I think your body is telling you there is something you need. I have developed a palate for fruits and vegetables as the main dish and not just something to add color to the plate. I have just enough fish to give me a week's dose of Omega-3, without poisoning me with mercury. I am not a vegan by any means. But I fill my appetite for meat with smaller portions and leaner cuts.

I am content with my abilities on the extension ladder; I stand upright and slowly find each rung as I pace myself. It is still not in my nature, but with forced forethought, someday it might become automatic. I kind of doubt it, after sixty years of racing to get things done. I pay attention to the tiny notes of wisdom my body gives me. My personality searches for humor in almost everything I touch. I have even been known to listen to my wife's advice at times. What more could anyone ask?

My mornings now begin with a handful of innocuous-looking, powerful pills. Oh, and of course, an alarm that blasts rock-and-roll with enough force to ripple the sheets covering me and Diana. So, I poke her gently between the ribs sixteen to twenty times, until she moans, gets up, and hits the snooze button twice to delay the noise for another ten minutes. The clock is supposedly a tool to wake her up. It's not. It's there to wake me up. I, in turn, am obligated to wake her up, so she can reset the alarm several times. The alarm and I work in conjunction to get her up for work.

She sets the alarm for seven a.m., but really, she wants to get up and be ready to leave for the day by nine. We usually listen to at least three sets of blaring music before rising from the bed. It is an absurd system, though it has worked for many years.

Of course, when I had to get up earlier than her, for the first fifteen of our twenty-nine years together, I arose within the first few bars that sounded from the clock radio. I got myself up and reset the alarm for ten minutes. She slept. The alarm blasted. She slept through the noise and the sunlight in an empty house. Then she called me later and griped that I hadn't awakened her. She was late many days and tended to rush, getting ready in a fifteen-minute tornado, a festival frenzy of clothes, hair curlers, and a blueberry Pop Tart.

For that reason, the mornings have always been a debate for us. I live with her system, but I hate it immensely. She refuses to let me use the water pistol on her in the morning. Diana seems to have no morning sense of humor. I wouldn't want water squirted at me either, but I'm not the one who has a hard time getting up. I'm just offering my services.

After ingesting my handful of cardiac-adjusting pills, I either swim laps or do "cardio yard work," as I term it. Cardio yard work is mowing, pruning, weeding, and watering. Most of my life I have avoided anything to do with soil, live green plants, and shovels. I now look forward to it in a limited way. I stand back and admire my handiwork, feeble as it may be. The swimming seems more aerobic. The gardening is more physical. Sometimes I do both. Both are invigorating and create a sense of accomplishment. Both are also tiring; but when I skip a few days of exercise, I feel the results.

It's interesting how some of the pills prescribed for me have taken awhile for my body to adjust to. Initially, certain pills affected me with face-flushing headaches, languorous movements, increased or decreased heart rate, overwhelming stupor, dizziness, a combination of several of these, or just plain left me sleeping in. I had to back off the dosages. There have been times I've had to call my doctor and have a completely different pill prescribed. I can usually take small doses, gradually upgrading, until I'm at the desired dose.

I once asked my cardiologist about taking so-called natural remedies, such as fish oil, Ginkgo Biloba, or vitamins. I didn't think I needed more pills, but my wife was enamored by the idea. She had been her usual, consumed, dedicated person, researching exhaustively on the internet.

Dr. Vandoven asked me, "Do you eat vegetables, fruit, and small amounts of meat? Do you eat whole-grain bread and cereal? And do you get daily sunshine by going outside?"

"Of course," I replied. "I can pass up fast food intercoms without many tears. Though there are times I have cravings and grab a cheeseburger and fries. My stomach and body usually regret it after, but it tastes great at the time. In general, yes, I eat a balance of the old nutrition pyramid."

"Let me explain it this way," he said. "Those natural remedies, taking up a whole aisle by themselves in the grocery store, won't harm you . . . for the most part."

He explained that most of those things are found in the foods you eat; in some cases, your body manufactures them. That was something I knew, but I needed backing from a professional to get my wonderful wife to ease up a bit. So, if one eats a well-balanced set of foods, they will probably receive most of the same things.

Dr. Vandoven then talked about natural remedies not being all that powerful for people with major disease. He explained that there were benefits to some of them, but they couldn't compare to the prescriptions. "Think of the natural remedies," his hands went up, wiggling two fingers to make physical quotation marks around the phrase, "as bullets fighting a war. With enough of them, they can fight the enemy. Now, think of your cardiac drugs as nuclear weapons. They fight the war with much greater force than bullets and have less chance of missing the target. You would need an exorbitant amount of Ginkgo Biloba bullets to amount to anything."

"And, they seem to be as highly priced as the prescriptions," I added.

"Exactly," he stated.

"But," I said, "I guess they could help psychosomatically, for some people."

"Are you one of those people?" he asked.

"No, I'm just thinking out loud about making my wife feel better. She is all for this stuff. I don't want to pop her bubble."

"You can take them if you want to," he said. "They won't help much, and they won't harm much. However, I should know what you're taking, in case it affects your regular heart medications."

With my impaired heart, food is a sedative. I eat and then relax while all that digestion goes on. I have found that my physical ability is hampered by all the blood needed to center on my stomach, letting it do whatever it does down there. It's simple; if I start painting a room or pulling dandelions from the grass right after lunch, I become dizzy, exhausted, and have to sit down. I have found it is easier to simply wait for a half hour or so.

After lunch and a digestive rest, I work on something. It may be cleaning a closet, trimming a tree, running errands, repairing a window blind in my wife's office, or all the above. It is a time of getting things done. My stamina usually lasts the rest of the day—until dinner, when my heart requires another digestive break.

Such is my life now. I had to take an early retirement because of my cardiac condition. I couldn't work the demanding hours my job needed. By the time I left full-time employment, I was completely exhausted and worn out. It took a long time to regain a basic degree of stamina.

There is no way of suffering through a cardiac arrest, or any other major health issue, without it changing your perspective on life. A person could become bitter, but I see no advantage in that. Most post patients I have talked to look at life and things around them with new fondness and find intrinsic value all around. They also have a blossomed courtesy toward others that comes from within. The world has greater wonderment. You feel alive and more sympathetic to others. You have a sense of happiness deep inside, knowing you were on the positive side of the 50 percent mortality rate associated with heart attacks.

These feelings and attitudes don't develop immediately. They are more like waiting for the hot water in an old home to stroll through all those copper pipes until the warmth of the hot water heater starts to trickle in, then streams from the tap through your hands. It takes some houses longer to build up the tepid water than others. Similarly, we just went through a scary, debilitating event in our lives. It takes a lot of clock-ticking days to resolve and process the initial shock. The dogma that "it happens only to other people" takes a while to wear off until a toasty feeling of content that we survived gradually absorbs us. Even if just for a while. Because, like all good feelings, it fades in and out, depending on all the other things life throws at us.

Life becomes precious, breaking down into each minute instead of days and weeks. It is full of amazement. It is almost sickening how grass becomes greener, trees fuller, grandchildren more cuddly, irritating friends and family more understandable, duties more enjoyable, work more rewarding, and time more inherently wonderful.

At this peak of new life, years after being a victim of near-death, it is an underlying awareness I have. Life is precious, slowing down to take notice is well worth the time.

I have found that certain foods twist my heart and my whole body, leaving me feeling like I've been in a car wreck. One of those things is sweets. I can eat a candy bar—but only if I do it in three sittings, taking about two bites per sitting. If I try to down a whole Snickers or Babe Ruth, I go into a toxic sugar rush. My heart beats too quickly, I get a slight shortness of breath, and I have to drink elephant-size gulps of water to dilute the sugar. That never happened with my previous good heart. I have never had what one would call a sweet tooth, though I have dabbled when the urge hit. Now, I can't even eat a whole Pop Tart, which is essentially a sugar-frosted jam sandwich. Why do things that are so bad for you taste so good? Or is it just the idea that they are somewhat forbidden?

I have mostly cut out beef. I find that when I eat more than a few ounces of red meat or eat it more than twice a week, I become lethargic, totally drained of energy. I'm not sure if it affects most cardiac patients or just me but think of the money I save by ordering petite cuts. Chicken and fish don't cause any problems, unless I overeat. But stuffing my belly with too much of anything causes me phantom pains and a day on the couch. Digestion must take a tremendous amount of energy and blood. At least it feels that way.

My heart has become an alarm when it comes to eating. My stomach has its problems too, but my heart tells me what I should eat and how much. I believe it is my body's defense to help keep a sickly heart from getting worse. I'm not sure this happens to all cardiac patients, but it should.

I visit my cardiologist every six months. The office hasn't changed in ten years. The fish are still swimming behind glass, displaying their colored stripes and dots as they dart and scamper and hide. I sometimes wonder if any of those fish were there during my initial visits. I have no idea how long tropical fish live. The rows of industrial seating and the tables littered with ripped magazines are the same each time I go. Magazines get updated but are never current. The receptionists vary. Most are young and go on to better jobs or to diaper-changing duties and dropping children off at school.

The nurse calls my name. I'm escorted in, weighed, and led to an exam room. She asks a few questions, takes my blood pressure, and closes the door on the way out. I wait.

Nowadays, there is a wonderful lady technician who begins my visits by checking my ICD. She sets a small, fat halo over the pacemaker and uses a computer and a mouse to run my heart through a myriad of tests. One test involves telling the ICD to race my heart several times. It used to feel as though I was at the end of a five-mile run. My chest would constrict and hurt. It was frightening to have my heart pump so rapidly. Now, after a few years with the device, it feels inconvenient, but not harmful.

The machine that checks my ICD spits out a few sheets of paper. The machine is essentially a computer, called a programmer. It communicates through radio waves, receiving and sending information to my ICD. The ICD tells it of any rhythm problems since the last checkup. The programmer makes adjustments, if needed. All my cardiac information is printed in graphs and charts on the paper. It is also sent through the computer system to Dr. Vandoven for him to peruse.

While the machine is working, the technician tells me of dates and times of problem occurrences since my last visit. Usually, there are only one or two. With my short-term memory stunted from my bypass surgery, I rarely recall any of them happening. I am not consciously looking for them, though. I assume if they are bad enough, I will know immediately.

My doctor enters the room shortly after my ICD technician leaves. He has obviously glanced at the report, skimming through the most pertinent information in the mass of electronic paper that shows up on his computer. So far, he has given me a verbal thumbs up. "Keep doing whatever it is you are doing," is the phrase that buoys me up.

We then go on to talk about medical advances or the book I'm reading at the moment or questions I have about some internet search that has caused me anxiety or a laugh. We have discussed the absurdity of heart transplants for me. There have been discussions involving the strides cardiac medicine has made over cancer treatments. We have talked about boating, waterskiing, stem cell research, alcohol consumption, the work I'm doing on my cabin, conservation in Africa, and limited amounts of politics. I don't recall ever talking about the weather. Thank heavens for that.

I always feel better after I've had my six-month checkup. I walk a bit straighter, chest out, with purpose. I have made it another six months on earth. The trees have leaves every spring through fall. I watch the sun glisten off them, then notice when their color darkens and the moonlight changes their sheen. I know I have taken fourteen breaths a minute through all the minutes of today, and it seems I have a good chance of repeating it all tomorrow.

There are times my mind thinks in terms of a mid-twenty-year-old, or other times a five-year-old, but my heart whispers in a low rumble then shoots wake-up tingles deep in my chest, letting me know I'm not. I cannot go back. There is only forward progression.

Regardless, it is soothing and substantial to watch the sun come up in the morning and the moon follow a similar path, then receive an encore over and over. Life is a wonderful thing.

But if you're at the bowl and your pee turns orange after a backache, watch out—you may have had a heart attack. If that's the case, try a little tea and toast. If that doesn't work, you had better head to the ER.

Remember, all through life's peaks and valleys, grow smiles and laugh with gusto.

Final Thoughts

Find what works for you. As much as all of us are very simular, we are all different. We all have varied likes and dislikes—things that can make one person laugh and another cry—things that boost your spirit on one day may cause anguish on another—people see things differently or they interpret them differently. Find what works for you.

Laughter and sarcasm and jokes and smiles are my remedy.

People cannot laugh and be angry at the same time. It's impossible to hold a grudge against someone when the two of you are giggling uncontrollably. Have you ever noticed how you can walk into a conversation and only hear the punch line, but you still howl with glee along with everyone else? You have no idea what the joke was even about, but you laughed. Laughter is contageous, just as misery is contageous. Find positive people to be around who know how to joke around with each other. People that don't mind a chuckle and even a snort once in a while. Even though you may be suffering an illness or a loss, it's okay to laugh once in a while. You will find the more you do it the better your life will become. Simple pleasure during trying times is not a bad thing. Break up. Crack up. Enjoy. As far as I know, you only get one chance at this life, and you should make the best of it. You can die laughing, but you can't actually die, laughing.

Going the other way—feeling bad about your life, your illness, your misfortune—only takes you down. The more you dwell on bad events, the further down you're going to go. Stop it! Just stop it!

Try smiling at the next person who passes you by. Guess what? Ninety-nine percent of the time they smile back. It also makes you feel pretty good inside. Think about something happy in your life or someone else's life or a funny thing that happened, and just smile. It's not difficult, even though it might seem like it at first. Habits are hard to break. You need to make smiling your habit. Try a little one day, and build on that. You will start to find more things to smile about. You can't form a whole smile—one that radiates throughout your whole body—and have depressing thoughts at the same time. A smile is a simple way to help you through those bad times.

Try listening to the lyrics of "When You're Smiling," sung by Louis Armstrong, and to "Smile though your Heart Is Breaking," sung by either Michael Jackson or Nat King Cole. That should help you put on a few extra grins through the day.

I don't believe my life was the most difficult experience anyone has ever gone through. It was far from that. Yes, I lost a son and gained coronary artery disease, but I have gotten through that and carry it as just a part of my life. I look at this whole set of events as horrid, but not as bad as it could have been. I've only lost one son. I broke the odds and lived through two coronary arrests. All the rest of my children are good and healthy at this time. I have an incredible wife who puts up with my shenanigans. I'm not exactly sure what shenanigans are, but I'm told they're extremly harmless fun. I have reasonable health. Sure, there are things I can't do and would like to do, but there are millions more things I still can do—like smile and laugh.

I have given much thought to things that turn bad things into better things—ideas that invert those diseased sufferings. I would like to give you a list I came up with and a few thoughts about each.

1.   Look for smiles on people's faces; better still, smile and wait for the return gesture. That single act relieves more pain than any other. You never know what anguish or unsettledness they have, but it's impossible fro them to not grin back even for a brief moment.

2.   Try to travel to somewhere new and different. When your mind is focused on the outside world and you actually see it for the first time, the colors are brighter and your thoughts are sharper. You may learn something, or it may just make you feel more alive. You don't have to travel

far. Sometimes a few minutes in the car to a museum or park you haven't visited is all it takes.

3.   Be creative. Find a hobby, make something, draw a picture, write in a journal (positive thoughts), or join a group that does something you're interested in.

4.   Physical exercise is one of the best ways to break from boredom, worry, depression, and laziness. The couch and the TV are not your friend—they debilitate you. Whether you go to a gym or take a walk around the neighborhood or raise your arms up and down for several minutes, do something. Do whatever you can and try for more each day. Tons of studies show how much mental problems can resolve or lessen from doing exercise. It makes me feel so much better.

5.   Spend time watching children. They are the true clowns of society. Children do amazing things. They know how to play harder and laugh harder than anyone. This should keep you smiling and laughing for quite some time.

6.   Try reading a good book with a real story and a plot. If you pick the right one, it'll be hard to put down. It fills time and makes you feel good.

7.   Do some kind of service to others. Help someone else in need. This doesn't mean giving people money, though it could if you have extra. It might be a lunch or a visit or helping them paint a room. Helping others comes back to you significantly. Do you remember that feeling you get in your chest when you help another? It's so worth it.

8.   Take time for something spiritual. Go to church. Pray. Seek spiritual guidance.

9.   Accept help from others. I still feel euphoric when I remember those people who brought me and Diana Thanksgiving dinner when I was expecting nothing.

10.   Try out something new. Play a flute or the piano. Paint a watercolor and then another—you're bound to get better at it. Take the time to study the Mayans or General Patton or botany. Learn to dance.

11.   Listen to music that gives you pleasure or makes you want to dance—and by all means, go ahead and sing. I

don't think anyone can dance and sing and be depressed. I sing all the time and hope to hell no one's listening.

12.   Finally, enjoy what nature has to offer. Use all your senses—listen to its subtle sounds, smell it, taste the fragrance of outdoors, feel the texture of leaves and grasses. Go to the mountains. Visit the desert. Check out a botantical garden. And spend time in your back yard or a nearby park. Nature invigorates me like few other things. There is an air that you breathe outdoors that is so welcoming and wonderful, and you can't get it inside buildings. It makes me glad to be alive.